THIRD EDITION

PASS THE MRCPsych
Parts I and II

THIRD EDITION

PASS THE MRCPsych Parts I and II

All the techniques you need

Christopher Williams
Peter Trigwell
David Yeomans

ELSEVIER
SAUNDERS

Edinburgh • London • New york • Oxford • Philadelphia • St Louis • Sydney • Toronto 2005

ELSEVIER
SAUNDERS

© 2005 Christopher Williams, Peter Trigwell and David Yeomans. Published by Elsevier Ltd.
All rights reserved.

The right of Christopher Williams, Peter Trigwell and David Yeomans to be identified as
authors of this work has been asserted by them in accordance with the Copyright, Designs
and Patents Act 1988.

First edition 1995
Second edition first published 2000

ISBN 0702028193

British Library Cataloguing in Publication Data
A catalogue record for this book is available from the British Library

Library of Congress Cataloging in Publication Data
A catalog record for this book is available from the Library of Congress

Notice
Neither the Publisher nor the Authors assume any responsibility for any loss or injury and/or
damage to persons or property arising out of or related to any use of the material contained
in this book. It is the responsibility of the treating practitioner, relying on independent expertise and knowledge of the patient, to determine the best treatment and method of application
for the patient.

The Publisher

Working together to grow
libraries in developing countries

www.elsevier.com | www.bookaid.org | www.sabre.org

ELSEVIER   **BOOK AID** International   **Sabre Foundation**

The
Publisher's
policy is to use
**paper manufactured
from sustainable forests**

Printed in China.

Contents

Contributors   ix

Foreword   xi

Introduction   xiii

Chapter 1 **Important practical and preparation issues**   **1**
             David Yeomans and Peter Trigwell

 - Structure of the MRCPsych Parts I and II   1
 - Applying to sit the exam   3
 - Preparation   3
 - Practice   4
 - Mental health   4
 - Getting ready for the exam   5
 - After the exam   5
 - References   6

Chapter 2 **Learning styles and revision strategies**   **7**
             Peter Trigwell and David Yeomans

 - Condensing information   9
 - Appropriate sources of information   10
 - References   12

Chapter 3 **The Part I and II MCQ exams (ISQs and EMIs)**   **13**
             Christopher Williams

 - The MCQ structure and scoring in Part I   14
 - What should I learn?   15
 - The MCQ structure and scoring in Part II   16
 - Preparing for the MCQ exam   18

- MCQ technique   21
- References   26

Chapter 4   **The OSCE – objective structured clinical examination**   **27**
Malcolm Cameron, Angela Cogan, Nasim Rasul and Christopher Williams

- Introduction   27
- The content of the Part I OSCE exam   28
- How the OSCE is marked   31
- Revision strategies for the OSCE   32
- Example OSCE answers   36
- Exam strategy on the day   41
- References   43

Chapter 5   **The critical review paper**   **45**
David Yeomans

- Introduction   45
- References for preparation   46
- Why has the College introduced this paper?   47
- Knowledge and skills for the CRP   47
- Techniques for the CRP   47
- Research methods   48
- Clinical relevance and clinical importance   50
- A comment on statistical tests   50
- Evidence-based practice   52
- Critical review paper: worked example   53
- References   57

Chapter 6   **The critical review paper – key topics for revision**   **59**
Catherine Keep

- Introduction   59
- Types of data   60
- Common statistical tests   60
- Definitions of some important statistical terms   62
- Screening and diagnosis   66

- Randomised controlled trials (RCTs)   70
- Case control and cohort studies   74
- Systematic reviews and meta-analysis   76
- Other types of studies to know about   80
- References   81

Chapter 7   **Essay technique**   **83**
David Yeomans

- Preparation   84
- Essay spotting   84
- Structuring an essay   85
- Worked example 1   87
- Worked example 2   89
- Self-test followed by worked example 3   91
- The role of the examiner   98

Chapter 8   **Preparing for the long case (individual patient assessment)**   **101**
Christopher Williams

- Preparation   102
- Predicting and practising cases   104
- Coming to the exam   105
- The clinical assessment   105
- Clustering questions   108
- What to do with the 'difficult' patient   110
- The vital quarter hour   111
- Structuring your presentation   111
- Preparing to present the case   112
- Presenting the case   112
- The differential diagnosis   114
- Investigations   117
- Management   117
- Prognosis   118
- References   119

Chapter 9 **Presenting the individual patient assessment (IPA)**   **121**
            to the examiners (Part II)
            Peter Trigwell and Christopher Williams

- Presentation techniques   121
- Difficult questions in the long case   122
- The five areas assessment   124
- Interviewing in front of the examiners   125
- The present state examination   128
- References   130

Chapter 10 **Patient management problems (PMPs – the clinical vignettes)** **131**
             Christopher Williams

- What are examiners looking for?   132
- PMP techniques   132
- Opening   133
- The middle/main component   134
- Ending and possible problems   135
- Example: treatment resistant depression   136

Chapter 11 **If at first you don't succeed . . .**   **141**
             Kevin Appleton

- Failing the exam   141
- Looking to the future   142

Index   **145**

Contributors

Dr Christopher Williams
*Senior Lecturer/Honorary Consultant in Psychiatry,
University of Glasgow, Section of Psychological Medicine,
Gartnavel Royal Hospital, 1055 Great Western Road, Glasgow G12 0XH, UK*

Dr Peter Trigwell
*Consultant in Liaison Psychiatry, Leeds General Infirmary,
Great George Street, Leeds LS1 3EX, UK*

Dr David Yeomans
*Consultant Psychiatrist, CHOICE, Clarence House, 11 Clarence Road, Horsforth,
Leeds LS18 4LB, UK*

Dr Kevin Appleton
*Consultant Psychiatrist and Director, Starfish Clinic and Education, Starfish
House, 47 Old Mill Road, Grey Linn, Auckland, New Zealand*

Dr Malcolm Cameron
*Specialist Registrar in Psychiatry, Liaison Psychiatry Office (outside ward 2),
Royal Alexandra Hospital, Paisley G12 0XH, UK*

Dr Angela Cogan
*Senior Registrar in Psychiatry, Lansdowne Clinic, 3 Whittinghame Gardens, Great
Western Road, Glasgow G12 0AA, UK*

Dr Catherine Keep
*Consultant in Child and Adolescent Psychiatry, Bradford District Care Trust,
Honorary Senior Lecturer, University of Leeds, Hillbrook Child and Family Service,
Mayfield Road, Off Spring Gardens Lane, Keighley, West Yorkshire BD20 6LD, UK*

Dr Nasim Rasul
*Senior Registrar in Psychiatry, Gartnavel Royal Hospital, 1055 Great Western
Road, Glasgow G12 0XH, UK*

Foreword

Candidates for the MRCPsych exam tend to be most concerned about the level of their factual knowledge. Before the exam they worry – "will this question come up in the exam? – what is the right answer to that obscure MCQ? – have I read the right books?".

But there has been a quiet revolution taking place. More and more the exam tests the set of abilities around "what makes a good psychiatrist?". There is a world of difference between having good factual knowledge of psychiatry and being a good psychiatrist. Knowledge of the subject is vital but it must be coupled with understanding and with the ability to communicate that knowledge to patients, carers or fellow professionals. Knowledge must also reflect an appropriate set of values.

The third edition of this book is timely. It does something quite different from presenting an up to date digest of the factual content of the exam. It does not provide the elusive shortcut to success but it does, in a systematic way, lay out all of the factors which contribute to passing the exam. Readers are introduced to the main components of the exam, how they can best prepare, what the examiners are looking for and how to best present their knowledge in whatever format be it essay or OSCE.

In my view this book is not only the best possible starting point but also an invaluable guide to preparing for the MRCPsych exam. The candidate who considers the format of the exam, their preferred learning style (whether or not to form a study group, whether to write notes etc.), what resources are available to them and how to improve their performance is the candidate who is likely to succeed. The exam tests a series of skills and it is the development of these skills, and in particular the key skill of effective presentation, that this book aims to help candidates with. It deserves to be widely read by both candidates and those helping them to pass the exam and I commend it to you.

Dr Joe Bouch, MBChB, FRCPsych
Consultant Psychiatrist, Glasgow
Associate Dean and Director of CPD, Royal College of Psychiatrists

Introduction

Clinical competence and passing the membership examinations for the Royal College of Psychiatrists are the most visible criteria by which trainees progress up the career ladder in psychiatry. Taking the exams is costly in both financial and personal terms. To pass requires very significant work and commitment.

In writing this third edition, we have fully updated and revised the contents of the book. We are pleased that the previous editions have been well received and have established themselves as commonly used preparation aids. In this new edition we have the opportunity to respond to recent changes in the examination structure.

In common with the previous editions, this book is not a 'crammer' book of key facts for the exam. If you are looking for a book containing facts and information then this isn't the book for you. You will find that very few factual pieces of information are presented. Instead, it will help you to present the information that you have learned elsewhere (whether from formal revision, everyday psychiatric practice or other sources) in a professional and structured way. Even very good clinicians with a strong factual knowledge fail the exams because of poor technique. This book will help you use your knowledge and experience effectively to enable you to pass.

We hope that you will find our book helpful. In producing any resource such as this, many other people are always involved. We wish to acknowledge the help and support of the various tutors, lecturers and examiners who have contributed to the development of the Glasgow and Leeds Examination Techniques courses and the associated books.

Finally, but most importantly, we wish to thank Alison, Amanda, Frances, Hannah, Andrew, Kate, Hannah, Rebecca and Andrew for their support and understanding during the writing of this book.

Chris Williams, Peter Trigwell, David Yeomans
February 2005

Important practical and preparation issues

David Yeomans and Peter Trigwell

Structure of the MRCPsych Parts I and II

Part I

To apply, candidates must have completed 12 months of full-time (or equivalent part-time) approved training by the date of the written examination. Full details of how to apply are to be found in the *College Regulations for the MRCPsych Examinations*.

> **The Part I Exam**
>
> The Part I exam currently comprises a written examination and an objective structured clinical examination (OSCE). The 90 minute written MCQ paper comprises 'individual statement items' (recommended time to complete of 60 minutes) and 'extended matching items' (recommended time to complete of 30 minutes). Candidates are required to pass this paper in order to proceed to the clinical examination (OSCE). The OSCE comprises 12 stations which are chosen with the aim of sampling across the range of psychiatric knowledge and skill areas as specified in the curriculum. Each station is of 7 minutes duration and candidates must complete all stations. Patients are played by role players who are given a detailed brief upon which to base their role. Candidates will be assessed by one examiner in each of the OSCE stations. A minimum of a grade C ('average') performance or above for nine of the 12 stations will generally be required to pass the OSCE.
> There is now no limit on the number of attempts that candidates can make at the MRCPsych Part I examination.

The Part II Exam

To apply, candidates must have passed or be exempted from the MRCPsych Part I and have completed 30 months full-time (or equivalent part-time) approved training. Full details of how to apply are to be found in the *College Regulations for the MRCPsych Examinations.*

The Part II exam currently comprises several written papers and two clinical examinations.

The written papers consist of two MCQ papers, a critical review paper (CRP) and an essay paper, all of which last 90 minutes each. The two MCQs are the basic sciences paper and the clinical topics paper. In each, it is recommended that candidates spend 15 minutes answering the extended matching items and 75 minutes answering the individual statement items. The essay paper lasts for 90 minutes and one essay out of three options must be completed.

The clinical examinations consist of the individual patient assessment (IPA) and the patient management problems (PMPs), each of these exams lasting 30 minutes. With regard to the PMPs, candidates will be presented with three vignettes (each lasting 10 minutes) and their answers will be marked by two examiners. All candidates sitting the exam at the same time will be examined against the same vignettes.

The limit on the number of attempts allowed for the Part II examination has been removed.

For more details see *College Regulations for the MRCPsych Examinations* which will be sent to you when you apply to sit the exams. The College revises the examination procedure at intervals; *it is essential for each candidate to get the most up to date guidelines.* One of the best ways to do this is to visit the Royal College of Psychiatrists website on the internet at www.rcpsych.ac.uk/traindev/exams/index.htm.

Not infrequently there are significant changes to both parts of the exam and it cannot be over-emphasised how important it is to obtain the up to date College curriculum in order to find out what areas of knowledge you will be expected to have. Surveys have shown that it is surprisingly rare for people to send off for this curriculum and read it once it has arrived.

Applying to sit the exam

Before taking the exam you will need to find two 'sponsors'. One must be your clinical tutor and the other a consultant who you have worked with for at least four months during the year prior to the date of application. The deadline for getting your application in is surprisingly early; you need to request the forms from the College several months in advance.

Preparation

Once you have decided when to take the exam you will need to work out a timetable for your revision. This can help you to identify what work needs to be covered. It will also help to keep you on target for the exam if you stick to your timetable. Most people assign a period of 2–3 months for revision for Part I, and 3–6 months for Part II. It is best to work consistently, e.g. two hours a night, but be flexible to allow for relaxation, on-call commitments, and other occasions. It can be helpful to decide upon a day each week when you will definitely **not** revise. Regular breaks help to maintain commitment the rest of the time.

It may help to structure your revision timetable by following the contents of one of the major textbooks. You will also need a checklist of the subject areas in the syllabus to ensure that you cover everything required. A useful summary of the key components of the Part I and Part II curricula is published at www.rcpsych.ac.uk/traindev/exams/regulation/curriculumSummary.htm.

Practice

An analysis of your learning style, as described in the next chapter, will shape the way you prepare for the exams. Practice is essential in preparing for each component of the exam. It is important to test yourself regularly throughout the revision period in order to get feedback on your performance. For Part I you will need to practice multiple choice questions (MCQs, including individual statement questions and extended matching items) and OSCEs. For Part II you will need to practice MCQs, writing structured essays, critical appraisal of literature (CRP), presenting reasoned solutions to patient management problems (PMPs) and clinical assessment and presentation for the individual patient assessment (IPA) exam. All these features should be built into your revision timetable as well as your learning of basic information.

Familiarity with the actual exam can only be gained through practice. Be assertive in your pursuit of exam practice. Ask senior colleagues to listen to your presentations and give feedback. Each person you ask will have a slightly different opinion on what is good and bad about your efforts. Practice will help you to build up confidence in your abilities before you enter the examination room.

Mental health

Examinations cause stress over an extended period. It is worthwhile considering how the process is affecting you. Do you need a break? What about a holiday or a night out? If you do experience exam nerves it pays to practice relaxation beforehand. Although some people have been known to find anxiolytics helpful, medication should generally be avoided as it may affect your ability to perform in the exam. Last minute revision is sometimes more of an anxiolytic than an aid to memory. Do it if you wish to, but a day of rest before the exams can also be helpful.

Getting ready for the exam

Get study leave arranged well in advance. Consider a revision course prior to the exam. It is often helpful to take a week off work just before the exam to do final preparations. Do not be persuaded to cover for an absent colleague at the last moment; you have spent too much time, effort and money to let personnel issues get in the way.

Find a decent place to stay before the exam. Do not skimp on last minute comforts, especially if you can claim expenses. Give yourself plenty of time to travel. It is better to arrive two hours early than two minutes late.

With good preparation you can feel confident that the exam is not going to bring up too many surprises and that you can comfortably cope with any that do arise. When doing the exam, although you will feel some anxiety, good preparation should prevent you being thrown off balance by a difficult question, or at least enable you to function on 'auto-pilot' until you regain your equilibrium. If you follow the advice in this book, you will have pre-prepared answers and answering techniques for difficult questions. You will know how to impress examiners by your presentation technique. You will know the ins and outs of the exam structure and how it is marked. You will know what is expected of you. All of this will help reduce your anxiety and improve your exam performance.

After the exam

Certain parts of the exam, such as the 'basic sciences' MCQ paper in Part II, leave many candidates feeling that they have probably failed (although many will actually have passed). These feelings may continue for some time. Try to avoid talking in detail to others about how the exam has gone, particularly during the breaks between the different written and clinical exams in Part II. Try to avoid too many 'post-mortems'. Going over your answers again and again in your mind and analysing possible mistakes is rarely helpful.

You have to wait a while for the results. A holiday away immediately after the exams may be a good idea. If you pass, well done! If not, then **try again** as many members of the Royal College have had to do before. Use the feedback from examiners and keep working on exam techniques. (See Chapter 11: *'If at first you don't succeed . . . '.*)

Key points
- Obtain and read the exam regulations and information for candidates.
- Understand how they apply to you.
- When you have decided to take the exam, send off for the application forms early.
- Submit completed forms, with the appropriate fee, in good time.
- Formulate a comprehensive revision timetable, including time off for recreation, etc.
- Examination technique can help you communicate what you know to the best of your ability. Think carefully about this aspect of the exam.
- Practice, practice, practice.

REFERENCES

It is important to obtain and read the following Royal College publications:

1. A copy of the *Inceptors Handbook* which includes advice on careers in psychiatry, details about the examinations, college structures and committee information.
2. *MRCPsych Examination Regulations*, available for download from http://www.rcpsych.ac.uk/traindev/exams/regulation/regulation.htm
3. *Past Papers in Psychiatry*, available from the Examinations Services Department at the Royal College of Psychiatrists.

   These can be obtained from the Royal College of Psychiatrists, 17 Belgrave Square, London SW1X 8PG, UK. Tel: (020) 7235 2351.

Learning styles and revision strategies

Peter Trigwell and David Yeomans

It is often believed that success in medical examinations simply depends upon the regurgitation of facts. This is not true. It is possible to know the facts of a subject very well and still fail the examination. You can improve your exam performance with good technique. Technique refers to your style of learning and preparing, and then of presenting what you know to best effect.

Consider the nature of your personal learning style. Different people have different preferred learning styles.[1] Some may have a

---

Preferred learning styles

Serialistic learning style:
- Follow a step by step linear progression from one item of information to another.
- Focus on only one aspect of the problem at one time.
- Focus on facts and logic.
- Tend to prefer a linear delivery of material (e.g. by attending a lecture or reading a textbook).

Global/holistic learning style:
- Readiness to think divergently.
- Examine several aspects of the current problem.
- Formulate more complex hypotheses.
- Make use of wider previous experience and link this to the new area.
- Tend to prefer use of analogies and links to prior experience.

---

serialistic approach and others a more global/holistic approach to learning. These different styles appear to be stable over time and are summarised in the box on page 7.

The following is a list of questions about learning styles. Work through it point by point; it is designed to encourage you to think about how you learn.

- Do you revise in a **suitable environment**? (quiet, warm enough, well lit, minimum of disturbance). How can you **improve** the environment?
- Do you **structure your learning**? (– according to the Royal College syllabus). See *Inceptors Handbook.*[2]
- Do you know what **sources of information** you are most comfortable with? This is likely to relate to your basic learning style.
- **How much information** can you take in at one go? There is no point staring at a book when your concentration seems to have gone. Taking a break will also allow consolidation of what you have learned.
- **How much repetition** do you need? Does it help to read several accounts from differing books, perhaps followed by a re-read of your own notes to fix those facts in your memory? Alternatively, are you the type of person who prefers to learn just one or two large and up to date books really well?
- Do you **set goals**? (– e.g. learn the components of the cranial nerves today and test yourself tomorrow).
- Do you **achieve these goals**?
- Do you **review your progress**? (– plan and write out a **clear revision timetable**, and try to stick to it so that you do not run out of time).
- Can you **prioritise**? (– learn the common things before the esoteric).
- Do you **keep the exam in mind while learning**? (– in order to memorise information in the style appropriate to the exam).
- Do you **use your daily work to help you learn**? (– reflecting on your differential diagnoses, formulations and management plans, and presenting cases under exam conditions).
- Are you **adequately motivated**? (– try to make this positive,

e.g. career progression or self satisfaction, rather than negative, e.g. because it is 'expected' by others and you 'should/must/ ought' to do it).

- Do you **use others to help you learn**? Do you work best by your- self, or as part of a group? Many find that a combination of approaches is most effective. Consider meeting once weekly for several hours with other colleagues who are doing the exam. **Study groups** like this may provide helpful mutual support as well as assisting with your revision.

Condensing information

There is a large amount of information to learn, particularly for Part II, and certainly too much to review it all in the few days leading up to the exam. A number of techniques are available to aid rapid review of key information.

Reducing the quantity of information in books/written materials

- Emphasise key areas of text (highlighters, underline, etc.).
- Cross irrelevant or confusing materials out.
- Add new materials to margins.

Make notes

- Relatively long (such as writing out many sheets of A4) or short notes (e.g. key words/bullet points) may be used.
- These can be used to either replace or supplement books.

Other aids to remembering

- Making lists of key information can help you to generate and impose a structure on what you learn.
- Consider reinforcing your learning by using MCQs or writing an essay to test your learning.

You may find that your ability to remember clinical topics/materials is enhanced by:
- Learning cases/management based around a clinical structure (PC/ HPC, etc.).

- Imagining or writing down details of a 'typical' case that summarises all the important principles of assessment or management.
- Remembering a specific patient who encompasses a typical or atypical presentation, assessment or clinical management plan.
- Using visual ways of summarising information such as Mind Maps™.[3]

Appropriate sources of information

Part I

Many people have found it possible to pass the Part I examination using a group of small books such as those listed below. These books are suggestions only, but reflect the sort of level of knowledge and understanding which are required for this exam.

It is also worthwhile reading relevant sections of the *British National Formulary* (BNF). This contains an up to date summary of current prescribing practice.

Suitable textbooks/Part I exam

- *Revision Notes in Psychiatry*[4] or *Core Psychiatry*[5]
- *Introduction to Psychotherapy*[6]
- *Symptoms in the Mind*[7]
- A basic psychology book[8]
- *ICD 10*[9]

Part II

For Part II you may need to decide early on whether you prefer to comprehensively learn a large, up to date text (e.g. *Companion to Psychiatric Studies*[10]) supplemented by some journal papers, or use a mixture of smaller books and rather more journal papers. Do not forget to concentrate on the main areas; these are often overlooked as people become bogged down in the fine detail of more obscure topics. Learn psychology[8] and sociology **early**. These are key areas, particularly for the 'basic sciences' MCQ paper, and they take quite some time to revise. You should try and avoid the (common) situation in which candidates try to learn these subjects from scratch with only a month or so to go.

Web-based resources

A number of web-based resources exist. Try looking at the following to see if you find them of help:

- www.superego-cafe.com
- www.trickcyclists.co.uk
- www.mrcpsych.com
- www.psychejam.com
- www.mrcpsych-help.com
- www.fiveareas.com (contains support lectures linked to this book)

– and also the useful article on how to pass the MRCPsych at http://careerfocus.bmjjournals.com/cgi/content/reprint/328/7450/207

They provide details of revision courses, book reviews, examination hints and tips, self-tests and other useful information.

Key points

- Passing the exam requires a clear revision strategy.
- Exam techniques can be vital.
- Think about the way you learn – is it as effective as it could be?
- Revise with the exam in mind.
- Use your daily work to help you learn.
- Leave yourself enough time to learn everything you have to.
- Learning facts isn't enough. Practice is essential.

REFERENCES

1. Flett A (1996) Student personality and approaches to learning. *Teaching and Learning Occasional Paper No 1*. Leicester University: Leicester.

2. *Inceptors Handbook*. This is available from: The Royal College of Psychiatrists, 17 Belgrave Square, London SW1X 8PG, UK. Tel: (020) 7235 2351.

3. Buzan T (2002) *How to Mind Map: The Ultimate Thinking Tool That Will Change Your Life*. Harper Collins: London.

4. Puri BK, Hall AD (2004) *Revision Notes in Psychiatry*. Hodder Arnold: London.

5. Wright P, Phelan M, Stern J (1999) *Core Psychiatry*. Saunders: Edinburgh.

6. Brown D, Pedder J, Bateman, A (2000) *Introduction to Psychotherapy. An Outline of Psychodynamic Principles and Practice*. Routledge: London.

7. Sims A (2002) *Symptoms in the Mind. An Introduction to Descriptive Psychopathology,* Third Edition. Balliere Tindall: London.

8. Smith E, Nolen-Hoeksema S, Fredrickson B (2002) *Atkinson and Hilgard's Introduction to Psychology*. Wadsworth.

9. World Health Organization (1992) *The ICD10 Classification of Mental and Behavioural Disorders*. WHO: Geneva.

10. Johnstone E, Cunningham-Owens DG, Lawrie SM, Sharpe M, Freeman CPL (2004) *Companion to Psychiatric Studies,* Seventh Edition. Churchill Livingstone: Edinburgh.

The Part I and II MCQ exams (ISQs and EMIs)

Christopher Williams

Written multiple choice-style questions (MCQs) are used in both Part I and Part II of the exam. The written papers in Part I and Part II contain two different types of question – individual statement questions (ISQs) and extended matched item questions (EMIs). Although both types of question are used in the written papers, they are still labelled as MCQ papers by the College. This chapter suggests ways of planning your learning with the MCQ exam in mind and also describes methods to improve your technique so that you are able to use your knowledge more effectively.

What are individual statement questions (ISQs)?

ISQs are a list of individual statements which the candidate must state are true or false. One mark is given for each correct answer. No marks are given for an incorrect or unanswered question.

Example
1) The mental state in schizophrenia commonly includes visual hallucinations. (F)
2) Cognitive models of depression apply predominantly to patients from higher socioeconomic classes. (F)
3) The half-life of fluoxetine is 92 days. (F)
Etc.

What are extended matched items (EMIs)?

In EMIs a series of 10 potential answers ('options') are provided. This is followed by a scene-setting sentence or paragraph ('lead-in'). Finally the candidate must answer additional specific questions by choosing the correct answer from the initial answer options list.

Example

Options:

A) Aaron Beck
B) Capacity to cope
C) Selective attention
D) David Clark
E) Reassurance seeking
F) Catastrophic thoughts
G) Hyperventilation leading to dizziness
H) Mental imagery
I) Paul Salkovskis
J) Safety behaviour

Lead in: A 25-year-old man experiences symptoms of panic. In the cognitive model of panic:

1) A clinical assessment shows that he fears that he will collapse and die. Which type of thinking style best summarises this fear? *(Option F)*
2) Who developed the cognitive model of panic? *(Option D)*
3) How is the symptom of holding on tightly to a shopping trolley whilst walking rapidly round the supermarket described? *(Option J)*

The MCQ structure and scoring in Part I

In the Part I exam the 90 minute written MCQ paper comprises 133 individual statement question (ISQ) items and 30 extended matching items. The examination is marked by computer and carries a total of 223 marks – 133 marks for the individual statements and 90 for the extended matching items. Combined ISQ and EMI marks are then converted into a score between 0 and 10 and a score of 5 or more is required in order to proceed to the clinical examination (OSCE). This means that you are competing with a pre-set pass mark rather than with other candidates.

Make sure that you understand the marking scheme. The exam is marked using a neutral marking scheme. This allocates marks accordingly:

- No answer or a wrong answer: 0 points
- Correct answer: 1 point

What should I learn?

Obtain and read the Royal College guidelines about the content of the exam. Both the full document and a brief summary can be downloaded from www.rcpsych.ac.uk.

> ### Part I ISQ contents
> The 133 ISQ items should be completed in the recommended time of 60 minutes. This works out as a maximum of around 27 seconds per response. The College has published a breakdown of the proportions of questions asked in a recent exam (www.rcpsych.ac.uk/traindev/exams/regulation/breakdown.htm). On the paper reported:
> - 29% of the questions were based on psychology.
> - 17% were on psychopharmacology.
> - 34% were on psychopathology.
> - 20% addressed clinical theory and skills.
>
> More detailed descriptions of the sub-types of question in each broad category are also summarised on the College web-site. Please note though, this is a rough guide only and questions on other areas of the curriculum may be included in the exams. The exact number of questions in each category is also likely to vary.

Part I EMI contents

The 30 EMIs are suggested to be completed in 30 minutes. No published information on potential topic areas is published by the College, however some sample questions are provided. A number of revision books are available to help you practise these questions and a helpful review is available at www.superegocafe.com.

The MCQ structure and scoring in Part II

In Part II, two MCQ papers are completed and address *basic sciences* and *clinical topics*. Each of the two papers lasts 90 minutes and consists of 165 ISQs (recommended to be completed in 75 minutes, i.e. about 27 seconds maximum for each item) and 15 extended matching items based upon five themes (recommended time to complete of 15 minutes). The examination is marked by computer and carries a total of 210 marks – 165 marks for the individual statements and 45 for the extended matching items. The combined ISQ and EMI marks are converted into a closed score between 0 and 10 for each paper, and then combined to give a total closed score for the two MCQ papers overall. Again, this means that you are competing with a pre-set pass mark rather than with other candidates.

Part II ISQ contents

The College has provided a breakdown of the ISQ questions on two recent Part II MCQ papers (at www.rcpsych.ac.uk/traindev/exams/regulation/breakdownbs.htm). Please note the breakdown of the EMI questions is not reported. For both papers, it is clearly stated that the proportions of questions is merely illustrative, and may change. Additional questions may also be asked as long as they are within the written syllabus.

Part II basic sciences paper

On the Part II basic sciences paper reported, 51 questions were on psychology [key topics included human development (15 questions) and behavioural psychology, including the description and measurement of behaviour (17 questions)].

Overall, 19 questions were on basic psychology and the social sciences (including ethology).

Another significant area was neurosciences with 34 questions. These were roughly equivalently split between neuropathology, neurophysiology, with 11 questions each, and neuroendocrinology and neurochemistry, with 11 questions between them.

Interestingly, neuroanatomy had only one question on that paper.

The remaining two main areas were psychopharmacology, with 22 questions, and genetics, epidemiology, statistics and research methodology with 33 questions.

No questions addressed medical ethics and the principles of law.

Part II clinical topics paper

The majority of questions addressed general adult psychiatry, 54 questions (33%) (including classification of disease, preventative strategies, presentation of illness and treatment, hospital liaison psychiatry, neuropsychiatry, medicine relevant to psychiatry and HIV and research). In order of frequency of question after this came old age and child and adolescent psychiatry with 24 questions each (15%). Addictions ,learning disability, forensic psychiatry and psychotherapy and psychpathology finally had between 13 and 18 questions each.

Preparing for the MCQ exam

- Produce a clear revision timetable in order to cover each area of the exam adequately. You will need to start your revision **well before** the exam if you are going to cover all the subject areas.
- It is often useful to go on a **revision course** at the very beginning of your revision. There are several advantages to this. It can help you get your revision going, boost your motivation and highlight areas of weakness on which to focus your learning. It allows you to realise the depth of knowledge that you must aim for and the amount of time you need to set aside for your revision.

Using MCQs to help you revise

Although there is no substitute for a thorough understanding of the subject matter, completing both ISQs and EMI questions can help you revise and learn.

- At the beginning of your preparation for the exam it is useful to spend some time **writing** some MCQs. For example, after completing a chapter of a book, try to write a few ISQs or EMI questions on the subject you have just learned. This helps to **re-inforce** and test your knowledge and will help **highlight** the kind of information which is amenable to MCQs. The questions are also useful for later revision. Some textbooks such as the *Companion to Psychiatric Studies*[1] have linked MCQ papers related to each chapter.[2]
- As you read through your textbooks, mark facts which are MCQ-able with a **highlighter pen**. The number of black and white true/false facts are remarkably limited. This will help you focus your learning.
- Remember that the information needed to answer MCQs is quite different from that needed to 'manage a patient'.

Using MCQs to help you learn

A large variety of MCQ books are available – some focussing on ISQs,[3] some on EMIs[4] and some on both.[5] Some of these are better (and more accurate) than others. Some books contain whole papers of mixed questions; others consist of questions organised by topic. Both of these formats are very helpful, but should be used in different ways.

- Make your revision more interesting by using MCQs. Some people find that when they continually revise a set of notes over a period of weeks they cease to take any new information in. One way of preventing this is to practise MCQs on each topic shortly after you have revised it.
- Remember that MCQ books and papers can help identify the sort of information which is asked in MCQ exams. **Improve your factual knowledge base** by reading and testing yourself with as many MCQs as you can. If you find you do badly in a particular subject or topic, target your reading towards these areas. You can then re-read the topic looking for the answers to the questions that you got wrong. This helps highlight particular areas of a subject as important, and allows you to add important details to your notes.
- Don't try to remember hundreds of dislocated facts. Instead try to **integrate** information you learn with your existing knowledge so that you **understand the principles** involved. **Summary notes** may help you do this. Of most value are those books which **explain** the answers so that you add to your knowledge.

Subject spotting

Exam courses often emphasise subject spotting. By analysing previous papers and reporting the apparent frequency of different subjects, it is suggested that it is possible to target revision at specific exam-orientated subjects. It is clear that there are certain core subject areas that you must know and understand well. For example, it can be very tempting for candidates approaching the exam to 'put off' revising psychology, sociology, human development and statistics. Try to avoid making the mistake of leaving these topics until just before the exam. These areas are large and need to be learned well. **It is not possible to revise them in only one or two days**.

Trust your 'feeling of knowing'

In the ISQs, one mark will be awarded for each correct answer and zero marks for an incorrect response. In theory, if you haven't a clue about the answer, a complete guess should have an equal chance of being correct or incorrect thus resulting in an average of 0.5 marks. The odds fall in the EMIs where in theory you have a 1:10 chance of randomly picking the correct option. However, by using logic and deduction, you can usually bring your choice on each EMI question down to one of only two or three options giving a 1:2 to 1:3 chance of getting the answer right, even when you are not completely sure of the answer. In practice, however, some people seem to be naturally better at answering MCQ questions than others and will score highly because of their ability to make a **confident calculated guess**. One area which has been researched is the 'feeling of knowing' that candidates experience when they read certain questions. When you do an MCQ paper, you will find that you either:

- **Know** the answer with a high degree of certainty.
- Definitely know that you **don't know** the answer.
- Have a '**feeling of knowing**' that the answer is correct, but are not quite sure.

In a neutrally marked paper you must answer all the questions; **don't leave any blank**.

> **Please note**: If you are someone who has a high level of confidence in your answers, and yet more often than not gets them wrong, this shows that you need to improve your factual knowledge.

ISQs: can you say 'no'?

Overall you should be confident about your 'true' answers; after all you are answering it as 'true' because you have seen or heard it somewhere before. It is much more difficult to be confident about your 'false' answers – the fact that you think that 'A is not a feature of B' may simply reflect that you do not know much about the subject! **Candidates are less likely to answer a ques-**

tion if the correct answer is 'false' than if it is 'true'. Therefore being able to correctly answer the 'false' questions can give you the edge over other candidates, and be a very valuable source of extra marks.

The confidence test

Complete several ISQ papers using your normal answering style. Repeat the papers after changing your strategy by answering more questions which you feel are wrong as false. Compare your marks with your usual answering style. **Do you gain or lose marks using this technique**? If you are consistently gaining marks, you should actively consider altering your threshold of response.

In addition, consider carrying out a more detailed analysis on your answers on several papers. Try to identify if there are **areas of knowledge** in which you have a particularly low level or high level of confidence (e.g. you may have a greater confidence in psychopathology than in drug treatments, etc.).

MCQ technique

Timing and practical issues

Check the up to date College examination instructions and regulations to find out how many questions you have to complete and what time is allocated. The structure and content of the exam may change.

- For the ISQ, **read each question very carefully**. Mark it as true or false.
- For the EMI, make sure you have read and understood the scene-setting sentence or paragraph ('lead-in'), and also each specific question.
- In the EMI, identify which options you can immediately rule out. Use your sense of logic – for example if a person's name is asked for as the originator of a theory/treatment, etc., the answer will be one of the surnames listed rather than a named drug! Even if

you then have to guess, you have significantly increased your chances of scoring a mark on that question.

- Have you understood the question? Anxiety can sometimes cause you to read the question cursorily and miss important aspects of the question.
- Be particularly careful with questions on topics about which you are confident. Your elation may lead you to misread the question and lose marks where you should have gained them.
- Make sure you put each answer **straight away** onto the **right line** of the marking sheet. Review this every few questions. It is easy to get your answers out of order. This will cause panic and could cost you the exam.
- Ruthlessly **skip** those questions where you really don't know the answer and come back to them later. You may find that other questions trigger your memory, and the answer will come back to you as the exam continues. If you still have no idea make a guess response. **Do not leave questions blank at the end of the exam**.
- Review your progress and maintain momentum. Remember that for the ISQs there is no more than 27 seconds available per question, so that in 10 minutes you need to have completed at least 24 questions, to allow for some review time at the end of the paper.
- Regularly (say every 10 questions), **check that you have transcribed the answers onto the correct line on the answer sheet**.
- Consider whether to stay in or leave the room when you have completed the paper. Many people benefit by staying and going through the paper one more time. **Again, make sure you have made an answer to every question**.
- If you are finding the paper horrendously difficult it is likely that others are too. Do not give up. Carry on and try to finish. Do not leave the exam hall in despair. You can still pass.

Don't be too clever

- Do not automatically assume that the examiners are trying to trick you. Avoid agonising over possible hidden meanings, as this is more likely to hinder rather than help your decisions.

- In MCQs, the 'correct' answer to a question is the **generally accepted version of the truth**. If you have some special knowledge of a topic that is at variance with the most prevalent view point – swallow your pride and save it for another time.

The numbers game

- **Don't waste time counting your answers**; you really don't know how many you have correct. Answer every question to the best of your ability.

Be aware of the techniques examiners use in writing ISQs

It is surprisingly difficult to write a good ISQ. Understanding some of the techniques used will help you to avoid some of the possible pitfalls. It is useful to think about questions from the perspective of the person writing them. They will wish to have a spread of true and false responses, of varying degrees of difficulty. Ideally the questions will be able to discriminate between those who know a subject well and those whose knowledge is superficial.

It is relatively easy to formulate 'true' questions. Read a chapter in a textbook and see how easy it is to pick out five facts that are true. The question can be made more difficult either by choosing obscure facts or by expressing the question in a form that is unlikely to have been read in a textbook, but can be worked out if the subject is known well. It is possible that you will sometimes know the answer to a question but not realise it. This is because the question has been **phrased in an unexpected way** or because it occurs in an unexpected place.

It is much more difficult for the examiners to write good 'false' questions. They may be created by using **popular misconceptions** or by using the **opposite** of the truth. The examiners will write the question by '*switching*' information that is found in sources such as textbooks.

ISQs: recognising the 'switch'

The following can be switched:

1. Nouns (or diseases).
2. Adjectives.
3. Negative to positive, or vice versa.

The wording of the question

It is important to look at questions from two perspectives: factual knowledge and logic. Good ISQs and EMIs are difficult to write and many questions contain some clues within the structure of the question. Use your common sense.

In particular, three commonly used phrases are:

1. A '**characteristic feature**' means that it is of diagnostic significance. Its absence might make one doubt the diagnosis. If it is truly characteristic then you are likely to be aware of it.
2. A '**typical feature**' is one that you would expect to be present. It is similar to 'characteristic'.
3. A '**recognised feature**' is one that, although it may not characterise a disease, has been reported. Marking this as false implies an in-depth knowledge of the subject, unless it can be recognised as a switch.

Other terminology

- ' **. . . is a pathognomonic feature**' means it occurs only in that condition. If you do not know the answer then it is likely to be false. There are few pathognomonic features and you are likely to know them.
- ' **. . . is associated with**' means that it is a feature which is well recognised but not common. The same applies to a '**. . . is a recognised feature of**'.
- Categorical answers such as '**Never, always, only, invariably**' should usually be answered as **false**, unless you are sure that they are true. Such absolute statements are rarely correct.

Use your sense of logic

The following techniques may help you clarify your thinking about an answer:

1. Look for terminology that is likely to make a question true or false.
2. Reversing the question (e.g. 'X **may not** occur in Y') can help clarify your thinking. Try this with some questions in any ISQ book to illustrate how helpful this technique is.
3. When practising, read the EMI question out loud putting each option in as the answer. Some will strike you as ridiculous and can be quickly discounted. Make your response from those remaining.
4. Look for items which are **contradictory** or the same. Contradictory items may be included in different questions later in the paper, and this can offer you additional clues.

It is important to remember that virtually none of the current MCQ books on the market seem to be as difficult as the Part II MCQ papers. If you feel that you have done badly on any one paper, **don't worry!** Firstly, self-perception is often wrong. Secondly, the marks on the two written papers in Part II are combined so it is possible to redeem a lower score in one paper.

Key points
- Make sure you know the structure of the exam.
- Start your revision early.
- Practise using a variety of MCQ books addressing both ISQs and EMIs and use MCQs to help you revise.
- Initially concentrate on a solid understanding of the subject matter.
- Start concentrating on MCQ-able facts at least 6–8 weeks before the exam.
- Work to perfect your technique.
- Read the questions very carefully.
- Don't panic: exam papers are often very difficult.
- Read the questions carefully, looking for clues in the wording.

> **Key points continued**
> - Keep checking your answers are in the correct place on the answer sheet.
> - Maintain momentum.
> - Using these techniques may help you gain some further marks, but there is no substitute for developing broad-based knowledge.

REFERENCES

1. Johnstone E, Cunningham-Owens DG, Lawrie SM, Sharpe M, Freeman CPL (2004) *Companion to Psychiatric Studies*, Seventh Edition. Churchill Livingstone: Edinburgh.

2. Johnstone EC, Lawrie SM, Sharpe M (2000) *MCQs for the Companion to Psychiatric Studies*. Churchill Livingstone: Edinburgh.

3. Mathews M (2001) *800 Individual Statement Questions for the MRCPsych*. Royal Society of Medicine Press Ltd: London.

4. Michael A (2004) *Get Through MRCPsych Parts I and II: 1001 EMIs*. Royal Society of Medicine Press Ltd: London.

5. Mahli G, Mahli S (2004) *MRCPsych Part I MCQ Practice Papers*, Second Edition. PasTest.

The OSCE – objective structured clinical examination

Malcolm Cameron, Angela Cogan, Nasim Rasul and Christopher Williams

Introduction

The objective structured clinical examination (OSCE) was introduced into the MRCPsych Part I in April/May 2003, replacing the long case. To qualify to sit the OSCE you must first pass the multiple choice paper.

The rationale for the OSCE is that it enables multiple skills to be assessed across multiple areas of working, compared to the previous situation in which a pass/fail decision was made on a candidate's assessment of a single patient – with history taking and mental state examination being the main skills formally tested. The OSCE aims instead to test a candidate's competence on day-to-day tasks such as explaining a patient's condition to a carer or completing a risk assessment.

The scoring is both structured and objective against pre-agreed criteria. This means that the importance of certain points in the history are decided in advance, and marks weighted accordingly, so candidates will be less vulnerable to the individual examiner's personal impression as to what they think is important.

All of this means the exam will be consistently set across different exam centres and also consistently marked. The impression of both examiners and trainees is that it is indeed a better test of day-to-day functioning as a psychiatrist.

The content of the Part I OSCE exam

The OSCE examination comprises 12 stations. Each station lasts for 8 minutes – so the OSCE as a whole takes 96 minutes. Candidates are given a pen and paper with which to make notes. Instructions for the stations are posted on the wall outside the station. The candidate has 1 minute to read the instructions. The instructions generally provide only a brief outline scenario followed by the task the candidate is to undertake. An example scenario is:

Example

You are asked to see a 40-year-old man who was involved in a road traffic accident. Find out what psychological symptoms he has as a result of the accident. (1 minute to read and plan your approach)

A bell will ring and the candidate then enters the station. You have 7 minutes within each station. On entering the station the examiner will ask you for your name and candidate number. From then on you will generally not be required to interact with the examiner again. The station will present a number of scenarios. Most commonly there will be an actor/actress who role plays a patient or carer. They are given detailed information to guide their answers so listen carefully to their responses to your questions.

There may also be some stations where there isn't an actor. There have also been stations where you communicate with a Consultant Psychiatrist (who is also the examiner for that station) over the phone about a patient you have assessed (most likely a patient assessed in the previous station). Sometimes, instead of an actor playing a patient, you can be faced with a dummy (e.g. at a CPR station) or a doll head (such as in a Fundoscopy station). It is important to treat these inanimate objects as if they were real patients. You can also be presented with a nursing kardex, blood results or a brain scan to interpret.

There will always be an examiner present. The examiners are themselves given little direct instructions but are given a mark sheet and for most of the stations have to assess the candidate in four or five areas (see the *'How the OSCE is marked'* section below).

The bell will ring after 6 minutes to warn you that you are nearly out of time. At 7 minutes the bell goes again and the candidate must stop immediately and go to the next station.

There may be a pilot station which is being tested for future exams, but this will not count towards your mark. There will also be a rest station. Excluding rest and pilot stations the duration of the OSCE is 1 hour and 36 minutes.

Contents of the stations

The content of each OSCE station will be a general adult or old age psychiatry topic. The subject of the stations aims to test a wide range of psychiatric knowledge and skill areas.

The following headings are a guide to the areas likely to be covered:
- History taking
- Mental state examination
- Communication skills
- Examination skills
- Practical skills
- Emergency management
- Miscellaneous

History taking skills may ask you to take a basic history from a patient with a mental illness, e.g. anxiety, obsessive-compulsive disorder, depression, memory problems or a drinking problem.
Mental state examination stations will test your ability to elicit symptoms from the MSE such as first rank symptoms of schizophrenia.

Communication skills are assessed throughout the OSCE and particularly in stations such as instructing a patient regarding discharge from hospital, consent to ECT or explaining a subject to a patient or to a carer.

Examination skills can be tested by getting you to examine a variety of systems, e.g. cranial nerves, a different part of a neurological examination, blood pressure estimation, fundoscopy, etc.

Practical skills such as application of ECT electrodes, ECG leads or CPR (resuscitation) technique may be examined.

Emergency management stations may centre on the treatment of severe drug side effects such as neuroleptic malignant syndrome or rapid tranquillisation of a violent patient.

Miscellaneous topics could include data interpretation, e.g. analysing blood results or interpreting an ECG or CT/MRI scan.

The commonest stations to date

The following are the commonest OSCE stations to date as identified by Glasgow-based candidates:

- Overdose risk assessment.
- Anxiety history.
- Cranial nerve examination.
- Eating disorder history.
- Psychotic symptom history.
- Cognitive assessment.
- Explaining ECT.
- Assessing capacity.
- Alcohol history.
- Explaining lithium treatment.
- Explaining psychological treatment of agoraphobia/phobic disorders.

How the OSCE is marked

Each station has predetermined objectives that the candidate doesn't see but are set out on an examiner's mark sheet.

Example

At a station where the candidate is required to provide an explanation of schizophrenia to a relative, the mark sheet may look like this:

Example OSCE mark sheet					
	A	**B**	**C**	**D**	**E**
COMMUNICATION					
NATURE/FEATURES OF SCHIZOPHRENIA					
CAUSAL EXPLANATION					
TREATMENT AND SIDE EFFECTS					
OUTCOME					
ISSUES OF RISK					
GLOBAL RATING					

The examiner awards an A to E on each of these objectives and provides an overall global rating.

Guidance is given by the Royal College of Psychiatrists that an average of C or above for at least nine of the 12 stations is required to secure a pass. There is however no single station which you must pass in order to be able to pass overall.

A detailed examiner's assessment sheet is available for download at http://www.prepdublin.com/Downloads/TRIAL%20MS2.pdf

Revision strategies for the OSCE

How to prepare
- Read the present state examination (PSE or SCAN) beforehand. This provides a range of useful questions and prompts for identifying the full range of psychopathology. Some examples of the use of PSE questions are provided in Chapter 9 (pages 128–129).
- Practise physical examination skills, e.g. how to assess all aspects of the neurological system.
- Practise with a Consultant during supervision.

Using exam preparation websites
A number of web-based resources exist. Try looking at the following to see if you find them of help:

- www.superego-cafe.com
- www.trickcyclists.co.uk
- www.mrcpsych.com
- www.psychejam.com
- www.mrcpsych-help.com

Some of these sites provide details of previous exam stations as well as numerous worked examples of model answers.

Detailed areas to prepare
Based on our experience of talking to those who have sat the Part I exam over recent years, it is worthwhile paying particular attention to the following areas. All have been examined before.

Affective disorders: assessment and management
- Basic history taking of depression and hypomania from patient or relative.
- Postnatal depression assessment.
- Abnormal grief reaction.
- Explaining to a relative the proposed treatment or illness/diagnosis.
- Psychological treatments of depression.

- Describing the need for/compliance with or side effects of antidepressants medication.
- Lithium pharmacology.
- Essentials of relapse prevention (e.g. Williams et al[1,2]).
- Medication adherence/concordance.

Anxiety: assessment and management
- Basic anxiety history to determine a diagnosis of anxiety disorder.
- Aetiology, e.g. role of hyperventilation, avoidance and the vicious spiral of anxiety.
- Psychological treatments, e.g. explain systematic desensitisation or an overview of the CBT approach.
- Biological treatments.

Capacity
- Key questions to test capacity.

Cognitive assessment and management
- Mini mental state examination (MMSE).
- Frontal lobe function.
- Parietal lobe function.
- Collateral information from relative on dementia.
- Assessing functionality of patient with dementia.
- Differentiating dementia from pseudo dementia.
- Cognitive enhancers.

Eating disorders: assessment and management
- Basic eating disorder history.
- Eating diary (use/rationale).
- Differentiating between anorexia and bulimia nervosa.
- Different reversing behaviours (e.g. abuse of thyroxine, exercise, laxatives and insulin).

ECT
- Explanation of procedure.
- Gaining consent.

Insight
- Important questions to test insight.

Premorbid personality
- Important questions to determine premorbid personality (from patient or carer).

Psychotherapy
- Explain CBT: essentials of model, key interventions.
- Explain psychodynamic psychotherapy.
- Key elements of problem solving (seven-step plan).
- Overcoming avoidance – for example in phobias.

How to deliver key CBT interventions are summarised in the five areas approach to CBT.[1,2] This includes both jargon-free ways of communicating the cognitive behaviour therapy model, and also a detailed and straightforward description of key interventions such as problem solving, relapse prevention techniques, etc. (details at www.fiveareas.com).

Schizophrenia: assessment and management
- Basic history.
- Explaining to a relative the illness/treatment.
- Eliciting first rank symptoms.
- Eliciting other psychotic symptoms, e.g. passivity, auditory hallucinations.
- Starting treatment.
- Treatment resistance.
- Extra-pyramidal side effect (EPSE) examination.

Substance misuse: assessment and management
- Basic alcohol history.
- Basic drug misuse history.
- Alcohol diaries (use/rationale).
- Advice on how to reduce consumption.
- Assessing motivation to stop drinking.
- Key elements.

Suicide/self-harm
- Basic risk assessment history.

Clinical examination skills

Practise and be able to do the following in a professional and confident manner:

- Examine the cranial nerves.
- Fundoscopy.
- Assess key extra-pyramidal side effects.
- Examine the thyroid (don't forget to examine the hands – warmth, pulse rate, and eyes – exophthalmos).
- Assess signs of alcohol or drug withdrawal.
- Test for cerebellar signs.
- Test for frontal/parietal lobe function.
- CVS/respiratory/GI examination.
- Neurological examination including tone, power, sensation and reflexes.

Practical skills

- Application of electrodes for ECT.
- Application of leads for ECG.
- CPR technique.

Emergency management

- Violent patient.
- Rapid tranquillisation.
- Neuroleptic malignant syndrome (NMS).
- Serotonin syndrome.

Data analysis

- Blood results, e.g. TFTs, LFTs.
- Neuroleptic malignant syndrome (NMS).
- Biochemical complications of an eating disorder.
- Interpret a CT/MRI scan.
- Interpret an ECG (EEG less likely).
- Analyse a nursing kardex (e.g. looking for any drug interactions or dangerous prescriptions).

Example OSCE answers

Example 1. Explain antidepressant therapy

Introduction

- Introduce yourself.
- Explain time constraints.
- Ask what questions patient might have about their use of antidepressants.

Discussion of principles of antidepressants

- Used to treat depression.
- Don't simply mask symptoms.
- Also used to help the symptoms of severe anxiety, panic attacks and obsessional problems; also people with chronic pain, eating disorders and PTSD.

Mechanism of action

- Neurotransmitters are the chemicals which transmit signals between the cells in our brains – chemical messengers.
- In depression, some of these neurotransmitter systems don't seem to be working properly.
- Antidepressants work by increasing the activity/levels of these chemicals in our brains.

Starting antidepressants

- Likelihood of side effects in the first few days.
- Latency of effect: that they may not feel better for up to 3–4 weeks, i.e. don't work straight away.
- Important to continue taking medication despite not feeling better in the first few weeks.
- Take them every day – or they won't work.

Explaining possible side effects

- Try not to be put off if you get some side effects – most get better in 1–2 weeks.
- Don't stop the tablets unless the side effects are really unpleasant, and if they are, make an urgent appointment to see your doctor.

Common side effects
- SSRIs – nausea, diarrhoea, headache, insomnia, short-term increase in anxiety, sweating, sexual dysfunction.
- TCADs – dry mouth, blurred vision, constipation, drowsiness, weight gain, tremour, sexual dysfunction.
- The list of side effects looks worrying and there is even more information on these in the leaflet that comes with the medication.
- However, most people get a small number of mild side effects which wear off.
- It is important to have the whole list so that you can recognise side effects if they happen.
- More serious side effects – problems with urinating, falls, confusion – are uncommon in healthy, younger and middle-aged people.

How long will I have to take them for?
- First episode – it is best for most people to continue taking antidepressants for 6 months after they are feeling better.
- For people who have depressive episodes over and over again, even when they get better, they may need to take antidepressants for several years to stop their depression coming back.
- Stopping too early is the commonest reason for people not getting better and for the depression to return.

Risks of suddenly stopping
- Discontinuation syndrome – stomach upsets, flu-like symptoms, anxiety, dizziness, vivid dreams at night, sensations in the body which feel like electric shocks.
- Most often with paroxetine.
- Can be prevented by slowly decreasing the dose of the antidepressant rather than stopping it suddenly.

Choice of drug
- Each patient is individual.
- SSRI or TCA depending on side effects, suicide risk, other supports.
- Other choices – NaSSA, NARI, SNRI.

Are antidepressants addictive?

- No – you don't have to keep increasing the dose to get the same effect.
- You won't find yourself craving them after you have stopped taking them. Discontinuation reactions can occur (describe briefly).

If I take them am I guaranteed to get better?

- Studies have found that after 3 months of antidepressant treatment between 50–65% of people who take them will be much improved – compared to 25–30% of those taking placebo.

What happens if they don't work?

- We can increase the dose and if no improvement try changing type of antidepressant.
- Adding lithium.
- Other treatments – counselling in mild depression, CBT self help (in mild to moderate depression), problem solving when depression caused by difficulties in life, CBT.

Example 2. History of memory impairment

Introduction

- Explain time constraints.

History of onset

- When did it start?
- What kind of things have you been forgetting?
- Gradually or sudden?
- Have things been worsening gradually or in a step-wise manner?

Other symptoms

- Any other problems?
- Changes in personality, e.g. apathy, disinhibition, irritability, aggression, accentuation of previous traits.
- Emotionally changeable.

- Episodes of confusion.
- Difficulty finding your way around, lost.
- Difficulty walking, falls.
- Difficulty speaking, finding words.
- Looking after yourself: dressing, washing, cooking, toileting, handling money, travelling.
- Insight.

Mood
- Ask about depressive symptoms including suicidality, self-harm, violence.

Hallucinations
- Ask about visual and auditory hallucinations.

Delusions
- Any strange ideas or beliefs recently.

Past medical history
- Ask about hypertension, heart disease, atrial fibrillation, myocardial infarction, peripheral vascular disease, diabetes, transient ischaemic attack (TIA)/stroke, epilepsy and head injury.

Drug history
- What medication are they on?
- Any worsening of memory symptoms because of anticholinergic effects?
- Any anti-dementia drugs?

Family and social history
- Family history of dementia, alcohol and drugs?
- Current social supports, empathy, how are they coping at present?

Example 3. Parietal lobe function

Introduction

- Explain time constraints.

Tests for dominant lesions

1. Finger agnosia

- Ask the patient to name/number individual fingers.

2. Astereoagnosia

- Ensure the patient's eyes are fully closed.
- Place various identifiable objects in the palm of the patient's hands, e.g. pen top, coin, key, matchstick, piece of cotton wool.
    - Ask the patient to identify the object using only sensory input from the hand and fingers.

3. Dysgraphaesthesia

- Ensure the patient's eyes are fully closed.
- Support the dorsum of the patient's hand and, using a suitable object such as the blunt end of a pencil, draw digits or letters on the patient's palm.
- Ask the patient to identify each in turn.

Tests for non-dominant lesions

1. Asomatognosia

- Inability to recognise parts of the body.

2. Constructional apraxia

- Ask the patient to copy the following shapes.

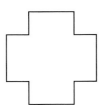 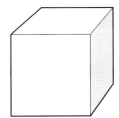

- Inability to recognise parts of the body.

Test the visual fields
- The optic tracts run through the parietal lobes to get to the occipital lobes.

Speech functions

1. Alexia
- Get the patient to read a short paragraph.

2. Receptive dysphasia
- Follow the command – 'take this piece of paper in your right hand, fold it in half and put it on the floor'.

3. Conduction aphasia
- Repeat after me – 'the orchestra played and the audience applauded', 'no ifs, ands or buts'.

Writing
- Write a sentence – isolated lesion indicates dominant parietal lesion.

Exam strategy on the day

Before entering the station
- Read the vignette carefully, not just one word and jump to conclusions (e.g. see the word 'alcohol' and assume it means 'alcohol dependent').
- Try and determine quickly what the station is trying to assess and what areas you should cover to gain marks.
- If you run out of time reading the vignette (they can be quite long), make sure you read the task you have to carry out. Remember there will be a copy of the vignette in the station if you wish to refer to it again.

On entering the station
- Introduce yourself and, in simple terms, your work position, e.g. junior doctor not 'SHO'.
- Describe the task you have been asked to carry out.
- Interact with the actor/actress not the examiner.

- **Listen** to the actor/actress as they have much more information to give if asked the right questions.
- Communication skills are important, even in the physical examination station.
- Don't write too much and avoid paying attention to the patient as a result. This is likely to irritate the examiner and probably the actor too.
- Stick to the task asked.
- Risk assessment issues are prominent in importance.
- Think of the whole picture (e.g. for a mother with postnatal depression you need to show that you have considered possible risk to the baby as well as to the mother).
- Remember biological, psychological and social aspects to a case (e.g. in the postnatal depression assessment mentioned above – is the mother able to interact with the child, play and smile at them? What impact might this be having on the child's development, and the mother's relationship with the father?).
- If you run out of time you can always say "at our next meeting we will discuss ….".
- If you have spare time or run out of questions, reflect whether there are any additional questions you should be asking. You can always summarise back out loud what the patient has said and check you have understood them correctly.

How to relate to the actors

You need to make sure that you maintain a polite and professional stance in your relationship with the actors. Address them exactly as you would a real patient.

- Check their name.
- Avoid jargon.
- Look for non-verbal clues.
- Conversation not interrogation.
- If you make a mistake, apologise and start again (e.g. rephrase jargon into normal language more understandable to the actor/patient).
- Thank the actor at the end.

> **Key points**
>
> - Few topics can be properly assessed using the OSCE format. Carefully consider what they might be and practice these assessments, explanations and practical tasks carefully.
> - The fact that frequency lists of previous questions are widely published is helpful – however it is only helpful if you can use this information to ensure that you are competent in each area. Rather than learning responses and assessments by rote, it is far better to gain a range of practical assessment and intervention skills. These supplemented by effective communication skills will help you present yourself and your skills well.
> - Avoid jargon and be professional in all you do.
> - Ensure that you practise this part of the exam. Reading can help but it is essential to practise completing the various key skills within the time limit available.

REFERENCES

1. Williams CJ (2001) *Overcoming Depression: A Five Areas Approach.* Arnold Publishers: London.

2. Williams CJ (2003) *Overcoming Anxiety: A Five Areas Approach.* Arnold Publishers: London.

3. Michael A (2003) *OSCEs in Psychiatry: Prepare for the New MRCPsych.* Churchill Livingstone: London.

The critical review paper

David Yeomans

Introduction

The critical review paper (CRP) is a 90-minute written paper which is completed in the Part II exam only. The paper is divided into two parts, one with seven parts accounting for 70% and the other with three parts accounting for 30% of the marks. Each part contains an abridged account of a research project and related questions. The questions examine your knowledge of research methods. You will be asked to critically appraise the studies presented. Some candidates report that they found it difficult completing the paper. It is important therefore to make sure you maintain momentum on the paper and complete as many questions as possible – leaving more difficult items and choosing to answer simpler and higher scoring questions as a priority.

Few exam candidates have become experienced researchers by the time they sit this paper. Their knowledge of critical appraisal is therefore theoretical rather than experiential. Fortunately there are many sources of basic advice on statistics and critical appraisal, and journal clubs should provide a forum in which trainees can develop their skills and confidence in this area.

This chapter aims to help familiarise readers with the aims and requirements of the CRP. A range of information about this paper and the syllabus and exam structure are available directly from the College.[1,2,3]

References for preparation

Unfortunately, no single book appears to cover all the knowledge and skills that are required for this paper. You need to be familiar with the basics of statistics and also understand the principles of critical appraisal and evidence-based medicine. The following list provides useful references for revision. These will help you become familiar with the language of research and critical appraisal and should provide most of the answers to CRP questions.

The books in references 8–12 will enable you to answer most questions; however no single book succinctly summarises all the terms and definitions required. Because of this, Chapter 6 has been writ-

---

Useful texts for revision
- *Critical Reviews in Psychiatry*[4] (Papers and mock answers from the College.)
- *How to Read a Paper*[5] (Critical appraisal methods.)
- *How to Read a Paper*[6] (Series of articles.)
- *How to Read a Paper*[7] (Internet versions of ref. 6.)
- *Statistics with Confidence*[8] (A useful book for understanding confidence intervals.)
- *Critical Appraisal for Psychiatry*[9] (Covers a range of key areas – evidence-based medicine, statistics, research design and critical appraisal.)
- *Evidence Based Medicine*[10] (Critical appraisal methods.)
- *Evidence-based Medicine*[11] (Detailed worked examples.)
- *The Pocket Guide to Critical Appraisal*[12] (Excellent description of critical appraisal.)
- *Evidence-based Mental Health*. BMJ Publishing Group, London. [Short format papers with critical appraisal commentaries. See BMJ website (www.bmj.com) for internet version.]
- Larger psychiatry textbooks also examine critical appraisal.

---

ten to summarise key elements that are important for the exam. Particular attention is given to the need to understand specific scientific concepts with a numerical value, and how to calculate them. These concepts have precise definitions and it will be helpful during your revision to build up a list of these definitions.

Why has the College introduced this paper?

The College wants psychiatrists to learn critical appraisal skills. These skills underpin evidence-based practice and the principle of lifelong learning. If you can read a paper and see its value, i.e. identify its good points and shortcomings, then you can assess that paper's relevance to your practice of psychiatry. You should make sure that your journal clubs become the main forum where you can practise critical appraisal skills with colleagues.

Knowledge and skills for the CRP

The syllabus and skills required are published in detail by the College. You will need to know about standard research methods. It is important to learn the advantages and disadvantages of the common types of research design. You also need a working knowledge of statistics. You must have an understanding of what standard statistical analyses can do and when they can be applied. Once you have appraised the methods and examined the analysis of data in a paper you should be able to assess the authors' conclusions. You should give a balanced answer, indicating strengths and weaknesses. At this point you can judge the relevance of the authors' work to your own practice and suggest ways of improving the design of the study.

Techniques for the CRP

You should start revision early. Critical review is a new area for many candidates, with an unfamiliar language. Not only are there novel ideas to learn in depth, but there are new terms to learn off by heart and associated numerical skills to develop. You will be expected to do calculations in the exam and you are allowed to take a simple non-programmable calculator in with you (make sure your calculator does not make beeping noises). Key terms are summarised in Chapter 6. You could compound errors too if terms such as the *likelihood ratio of a positive result* are calculated from the formula:

$$\frac{\text{sensitivity}}{(1-\text{specificity})}$$

– and you have previously calculated one of these values incorrectly. Early revision will give you time to familiarise yourself with the language of critical appraisal and practise the techniques.

Ring up for the College's information pack, sample papers and exam guidelines. Get a book of sample papers and answers to practise with. After your first attempt at a mock paper, make an assessment of your current abilities in critical review and begin to define the gaps in your knowledge. You can learn techniques for calculations such as the 2 × 2 table for screening test results (see worked example) which minimises confusion. Practise interpreting data in terms of the analytical definitions and calculations, e.g. *'How good is this anxiety test at picking out true cases?'* is the same as asking *'What is this anxiety test's sensitivity?'*, which is, numerically:

$$\frac{(\text{test positive true cases})}{(\text{true cases})}$$

Research methods

Different questions require different research methods. You need to know which method is best suited to each question. If you want to make conclusions about causation in the case of long-term exposure to environmental agents, you will need a different method to that used in assessing the effectiveness of a sleeping tablet. A description of the main research methods and common errors that may occur in research methodology are provided in Chapter 6.

You should be able to answer the following questions about any paper:

- Is the question relevant?
- Is the sampling satisfactory?
- Is the method appropriate to answer the question?
- Is the analysis appropriate and accurate?
- Are the results valid and reproducible?
- Has the question been answered definitively?
- Were there funding or ethical conflicts?
- Can and should I apply the findings in practice? Are the results generalisable?

The sampling procedure (and in particular whether the sample obtained is representative of the target population) is a key question. This is described in detail in Chapter 6.

Important questions to consider in your appraisal

- What about the setting? Researchers in tertiary referral centres are unlikely to see the same patients as someone working within an inner city psychiatric sector.
- What about the selection of patients? What about exclusions/inclusions? How representative are they of the target population?
- How would you improve on the design?
- Are other methods of analysis indicated? Was the correct analysis carried out?
- Are missing patients properly accounted for (see CONSORT guidelines in Chapter 6).
- How would you address the limitations of this study in future work?

Be prepared to extend your criticism into positive steps towards more accurate studies and more definitive results.

Clinical relevance and clinical importance

Just because something is statistically significant does not mean that it is clinically important. Here is a list of the type of questions you may be asked about the paper under scrutiny:

- How would you use the results?
- How would you explain them to your patient?
- Would you use this drug? Is it safe?
- Would this test be applicable in a different setting (community/clinic/hospital)?
- Would you withdraw this treatment?

You can only answer such questions in an evidence-based fashion after critically appraising the type of study, the methods, analyses and strength of conclusions.

A comment on statistical tests

You need to know about the different forms of data such as **categorical** or **nominal** classifications (e.g. male or female). **Ordinal** data can be ranked in order of size (i.e. ordered). A regular scale, such as centigrade, uses **interval** data. **Ratio** data have both a regular scale and also a true zero point (e.g. height in centimetres or temperature in degrees Kelvin).

Descriptive statistics

These include measures of central tendency such as the **mean** (average), **median** (middle value) and **mode** (most common result). Measures of spread include the **variance** (the mean of the sum of the squares of the difference from the mean), the **standard deviation** (the square root of the variance) and the **range** (the difference between the top and the bottom values). Measures of spread may have complex looking formulae which serve to turn inconvenient negative values into positive ones (by squaring them) and then make up for that by 'square rooting' them again. Details can be found in any book on statistics.

The type of data distribution in your target population (not your sample population) determines which statistical tests you should use. When your target population data are evenly spread around the mean and the mean, median and mode are equal, the distribution curve is bell-shaped, and the distribution is called **normal** or **Gaussian**. This distribution has specific *parameters* and the statistics used when analysing data with such a distribution are called **parametric**. Examples of normal distributions are height and weight in the general population. Non-normal or skewed data have asymmetrical distribution curves with unequal mean, median and mode. The significance tests for these populations do not have normal parameters and are called **non-parametric** or distribution-free tests.

Analytic statistics

Parametric statistics for normal data come in various forms. The simplest is the *t*-test. This can be an unpaired test for unrelated samples or a paired test if the samples are closely linked in some way (e.g. before and after comparisons on the same subjects). The test can be one- or two-tailed depending on whether you are interested in results in one or two directions. If you are only looking at the improvement brought about by a drug a one-tailed test is used, but if you want to examine improvement and deterioration, a two-tailed test would be appropriate. The *t* values can be looked up in tables which give probabilities (*p*-values) based on the sample size minus 1 (*n*–1) or **degrees of freedom**.

Non-parametric statistics include the Chi-squared test for categorical data, Mann-Whitney U test for ordinal data and Wilcoxon tests. These are used for non-normal data and small samples. They tend to give less significant results than parametric tests and are often based on ranking of ordered data. It is tempting to use parametric statistics in preference to non-parametric, but if sample sizes are small or unlikely to be from a normally-distributed target population, parametric analysis would be inappropriate. Some researchers will **transform** their skewed data with a mathematical function, such as logarithms, to get around this.

Confidence intervals

These indicate the precision of the statistic calculated. They give a range rather than a cut-off. Confidence intervals (CIs) are like goal posts. If the goalkeeper is the calculated statistic, then the narrower the goal posts (CIs), the more confident you can be about the goalkeeper's effectiveness (i.e. to represent the true population value). Confidence intervals can be calculated for most statistics and are commonly used with sample means. For example, if you were comparing the average values of depression scale results in two samples and you calculated that the 95% CI of the difference in sample means of 10 was 5–15, this means that:

- there is a 95% chance that 5–15 includes the target population difference of means; or in more practical terms:
- 95% of identical studies would have a difference of means in the range 5–15.

Small samples with more spread (bigger standard errors) have wider confidence intervals and therefore give less precise results.

Evidence-based practice

There is little evidence yet that evidence-based medicine is widespread. Few practitioners, for example, have routinely changed their practice in response to the NICE or SIGN guideline reviews. A survey of 24 general practitioners revealed that they did not share the basic assumptions of evidence-based medicine and did not practise evidence-based medicine because of patient factors (co-morbidity and non-compliance) and lack of time, resources and skills. Observation of hospital specialist practice was just as likely to bring about changes of practice.[13] It may be reassuring to know that medical colleagues find critical appraisal difficult, but it also suggests that we should be as up to date as possible since, as specialists, we will be influencing the practice of others.

Critical review paper: worked example

Critical review can seem quite daunting. The worked example is also demanding and so a light-hearted scenario has been created to finish off this chapter.

Question

The examinations department recognised towards the end of the twentieth century that its examination system was causing candidates so much anxiety that a less stressful alternative was needed. Feedback from trainees highlighted the problems, which included months spent in revision, sleepless nights in the week before examinations and profound gastrointestinal upsets on examination days.

After much debate the examinations department piloted a controversial new assessment based on the work of Rorschach which was first published in 1921. During a period of intensive research into early versions of the new assessment, candidates were sent four Rorschach inkblots and asked to jot down their general impressions of the images and return these in pre-paid envelopes. This paper reports a comparison of the inkblot results with the traditional exam results.

The results are presented here in a 2 × 2 table with the inner cells labelled by letter and the outer (totals) cells by letter sums. These are used in the calculation of test characteristics below. [Data are unlikely to be presented quite so helpfully in the exam but these tables can be constructed from the raw data of any dichotomous test that is compared with a dichotomous gold standard.]

		Traditional (gold standard) exam result		
		Pass	Fail	Totals
Results of inkblot test	Pass	a 82	b 93	$a+b = 175$
	Fail	c 7	d 18	$c+d = 25$
	Totals	$a+c = 89$	$b+d = 111$	$a+b+c+d = 200$

1. Comment on the rationale and methodology for this research.
2. (a) How good is the new assessment at identifying candidates who have passed the traditional exam? What is this aspect of a test called? Give its value.
   (b) How well does the new assessment identify candidates who have failed the traditional exam? What is this feature of a test called? Give its value.
3. Calculate the positive and negative predictive values and comment on the results.
4. What is the likelihood ratio for a positive result (i.e. a pass)?
5. Compare pre-test odds with post-test odds. (Alternatively compare pre- and post-test probabilities.)
6. Should the new test be introduced?

Answers

1. The research aims to find a satisfactory and less stressful alternative to the traditional examination. The new assessment is compared with the gold standard of the existing examination. The inkblot test is an observer-rated projective personality test. It is unlikely to measure the same things as the traditional exam. The test is subject to age, gender and cultural bias. No details of the method of interpretation are given. It is likely that the interpretation is qualitative rather than quantitative and inter-rater reliability between interpretations will be low. The omission of the methodology is a grave shortcoming in this research which means all the results are questionable. A 100% return rate is an excellent response rate and may be too good to be true.
2. The 2 × 2 table can be re-worked as:

		Traditional (gold standard) exam result			
		Pass	Fail	Totals	
Results of inkblot test	Pass	*a* 82	*b* 93	*a+b* = 175	**Positive predictive value = *a/(a+b)***
	Fail	*c* 7	*d* 18	*c+d* = 25	**Negative predictive value = *d/(c+d)***
	Totals	*a+c* = 89	*b+d* = 111	*a+b+c+d* = 200	
		Sensitivity = *a/(a+c)*	**Specificity = *d/(b+d)***		**Prevalence =*(a+c)/(a+b+c+d)***

(a) The test is good at identifying traditional exam passes. This aspect of a test is called the sensitivity. The proportion of traditional exam passes (gold standard) which are also new assessment passes is 92% (***a/(a+c)*** = 82/89).

(b) The test is poor at identifying candidates who failed the traditional exam. This feature of a test is called the specificity. The proportion of traditional exam failures which are also new assessment failures is 16% (***d/(b+d)*** = 18/111).

3. The positive predictive value is 47% (***a/(a+b)*** = 82/175). This is the proportion of new assessment passes which are also traditional exam passes. The negative predictive value is 72% (***d/(c+d)*** = 18/25). The new assessment is not a good indicator of the gold standard pass rate but is better at indicating a gold standard failure. (It is worth remembering that the positive predictive value is the same as the post-test probability of a pass).

4. The likelihood ratio for a pass is 1.1 (sensitivity/(1–specificity) = 0.92/(1–0.16)). The more extreme the likelihood ratio, the more useful the test. The least helpful tests have likelihood ratios of 1.

5. Pre-test odds = prevalence/(1–prevalence). The prevalence of gold standard passes is 45% (***(a+c)/(a+b+c+d)*** = 89/200). The pre-test odds are

therefore 0.82 (0.45/0.55). Post-test odds = pre-test odds × likelihood ratio, which is 0.9 (0.82 × 1.1). The odds can be converted to probabilities with the formula: odds/(1+odds). So pre-test probability is 45% (0.82/1.82) and post-test probability is 47% (0.9/1.9) (which is the same as positive predictive value, above). The test gives us no further information than the prevalence alone and is therefore unhelpful.

6. The methodology is unclear and likely to be subject to many forms of bias. The results of the analysis are suspect. The neutral likelihood ratio suggests the test would be unhelpful. The traditional exam has considerable face validity in that it examines candidates in the clinical process of history taking, mental state examination and clinical decision making, as well as theoretical background. The new assessment has no face validity and no theoretical rationale is given for the choice of the inkblot method. The new assessment should not be introduced and the traditional system with all its attendant stresses for candidates should be retained.

Key points
- Start revision and mock papers early on in Part II preparation.
- Use journal clubs to practise critical appraisal.
- Collect together books and other resources to help you learn and revise.
- Create your own list of definitions and calculation formulae. **Use Chapter 6 to help you with this**.
- Learn about research methods, analyses and statistics.
- Get used to applying research to clinical practice.
- Maintain momentum in the paper and make sure you pick up 'easy' marks quickly. Some candidates find it hard to finish the paper due to time constraints.

REFERENCES

1. *MRCPsych Part II Examination Guidance Notes.* Royal College of Psychiatrists, 17 Belgrave Square, London SW1X 8PG, UK. Tel: (020) 7235 2351.

2. *The Critical Review Paper Information Pack.* Royal College of Psychiatrists, 17 Belgrave Square, London SW1X 8PG, UK. Tel: (020) 7235 2351.

3. *The Basic Sciences and Clinical Curricula for the MRCPsych Examinations.* Royal College of Psychiatrists, 17 Belgrave Square, London SW1X 8PG, UK. Tel: (020) 7235 2351.

4. Brown T, Wilkinson G (2000) *Critical Reviews in Psychiatry,* Second Edition. Gaskell: London.

5. Greenhalgh T (1997) *How to Read a Paper.* BMJ Publishing Group: London.

6. Greenhalgh T (1997) How to read a paper. *British Medical Journal* 315: 243.

7. Greenhalgh T (1997) How to read a paper. Electronic *British Medical Journal* (www.bmj.com) 315: 243.

8. Altman D, Machin D, Bryant T, Gardner M (2000) *Statistics with Confidence,* Second Edition. BMJ Books: London.

9. Lawrie S, McIntosh A, Rao S (2000) *Critical Appraisal for Psychiatry.* Churchill Livingstone: London.

10. Sackett DL, Scott W, Richardson MD, Rosenberg W, Haynes RB (1996) *Evidence Based Medicine.* Churchill Livingstone: London.

11. Friedland DJ et al (1998) *Evidence-based Medicine.* Appleton & Lange: Stamford.

12. Crombie IK (1996) *The Pocket Guide to Critical Appraisal.* BMJ Books: London.

13. Tomlin Z, Humphrey C, Rogers S (1999) General practitioners' perceptions of effective health care. *British Medical Journal* 318: 1532–1535.

The critical review paper – key topics for revision

Catherine Keep

Introduction

> **Chapter outline**
> This chapter will summarise:
> - Types of data.
> - Common statistical tests.
> - Definitions of some important statistical terms.
> - Screening and diagnosis.
> - Randomised controlled trials (RCTs).
> - Case control/cohort studies.
> - Systematic reviews and meta-analysis.

Candidates approaching the critical review paper need to know and understand the key concepts of how to carry out effective critical appraisal. The concepts of critical appraisal are summarised in a number of good books (e.g. Crombie,[1] Lawrie et al[2]). However, many of the key statistical concepts required are not covered well from any one source and are therefore particularly difficult to learn for the purpose of the exam. This chapter is not meant to be a comprehensive account of all that is required for the critical review paper; however, it does aim to provide explanations and definitions for some of the terms and phrases that candidates often have difficulty with. Basic statistics (e.g. calculating the mean, median and mode) have not been included. A clear description of these and more advanced tests can be found within many different statistics books such as those recommended in Chapter 5. It is important to realise that learning these definitions by rote is not enough. You must attempt to **understand** these concepts which are drawn from the fields of research design and methodology, statistics and critical appraisal. Read about the different definitions and terms using different sources and practise applying them to the papers that you read in order to reinforce your learning.

Types of data

Type of data	Nominal	Ordinal	Interval	Ratio
Categories mutually exclusive	×	×	×	×
Categories logically ordered		×	×	×
Equal distance between adjacent categories			×	×
True zero point				×

Common statistical tests

Descriptive statistics

Mean, standard deviation. Median, mode, range.

Analytical statistics

	Parametric	Non-parametric
Comparison of two groups	Students *t*-test (paired or independent/unpaired)	a) Two independent groups: Mann-Whitney U Test b) Paired data: Wilcoxon rank sum test
Compare a large number of groups	ANOVA	Kruskal-Wallis ANOVA
Correlation coefficients (looking for an association between two variables)	Pearson correlation coefficient	Spearman rank correlation coefficient
Multivariate analysis	MANOVA Multiple regression Logistic regression	

Standard deviation
- The spread of all the observations around the mean.
- Calculated as *square root of the variance.*
- Have the same units as the original observations.

$$sd = \sqrt{\Sigma \frac{(x - \bar{x})^2}{n - 1}}$$

sd = the square root of the variance, hence the variance = sd^2.
- In a normal (Gaussian) distribution:

> 67% of the values lie between +/– 1 sd
> 95% of the values lie between +/– 2 sd
> 99% of the values lie between +/– 3 sd

Standard error
The standard error = standard deviation/$\sqrt{n}$ and hence includes a measure of sample size.

- It reflects the variability of the mean of the sample as an estimate of the true mean of the general population from which the sample was taken.

ANOVA (analysis of variance)
- Compares the variability of observations around the mean within a group to the variability between group means.
- Can identify big differences but not where they lie.
- Needs further post-hoc tests to identify where these differences lie (e.g. *t*-tests; Scheffe test to examine the possible combinations of group means).

Correlation coefficients
- Degree of annotation/association between observations. Rated 0 = no association, to 1 (or –1), directly (or inversely) associated.
- Describe average relationships.
- Cannot discuss cause and effect (e.g. smoking and lung cancer).
- Prone to confounding – other factors may have led to the finding.

Multiple regression

- A measure of association is calculated taking a number of con-founders (e.g. age, sex) into account simultaneously.
- A form of multivariate analysis.
- Applies when the dependent variable is continuous.

Logistic regression

- Used when the dependent variable is binary/dichotomous.
- The risk of developing an outcome is expressed as a function of independent predictor variables.
- The dependent variable is defined as **the natural log of the odds of the disease**.
- Can be converted to an odds ratio (see later) that is adjusted for confounding and/or into '**product terms**' to assess interactions.

Cox-proportional hazards/regression

- A method for modelling time-to-event data. The Cox regression allows you to include predictor variables (covariates) in your models (e.g. '*Do men and women have different risks of develop-ing lung cancer based on cigarette smoking?*'). By constructing a Cox regression model with cigarette usage (cigarettes smoked per day) and gender entered as covariates, you can test hypotheses regarding the effects of gender and cigarette usage on time-to-onset for lung cancer. (Definition and example taken from SPSS for Windows.)
- Includes a time factor – appropriate if subjects have not been fol-lowed up for an equal length of time.
- Another statistical approach used within survival analysis is the **Kaplan Meier survival analysis**.

Definitions of some important statistical terms

Target population

- The target population makes up a large pool of information from which we draw a proportion for study (sample population, see below). It will contain every eligible person or item having the characteristics of interest.

Sample population

- The sample population is a collection of individuals or items taken from a target population. The aim is for the sample population to be **representative** of the target population so that any conclusions drawn from the sample population can have **validity** and **generalisability**. Methods of sampling include random sampling, stratified random sampling, multi-stage random sampling and cluster sampling. Badly chosen samples can result in **selection bias**.

Null hypothesis

- The null hypothesis (sometimes called H_0) assumes that there is no effect (no difference) between the experimental and control groups, i.e. the data have come from a chance-based distribution.
- This contrasts with the experimental hypothesis (H_1) that assumes there is a true difference between the groups that has **not** arisen by chance.

Statistical significance

- Conventionally used to indicate the likelihood of a result as, or more, extreme than what is found, had it been drawn from a chance-based distribution (i.e. the probability of it occurring by **chance**).

p value

- If the null hypothesis were true, p is the probability of getting your result or a more extreme value by chance.
- If p is very small (conventionally taken as $p \leq 0.05$ or smaller), any difference observed is judged to have been unlikely to have occurred by chance. Thus the null hypothesis can be rejected – there **is** a difference between groups.

Clinical significance

Just because a result is statistically significant does not mean that the difference observed is of sufficient magnitude to be apparent and important in a **clinical** setting, i.e. is it of **clinical significance** rather than merely statistical significance?

Confidence intervals (CIs)

- The range of values within which we can be 95% sure (or whatever CI level is chosen) that the true value lies for the target population from whom the study patients were selected.
- If a series of identical studies were carried out repeatedly on different samples from the same population, then 95% results would lie between these values.
- Tells us about the strength of the evidence rather than if there is just a difference.
- It provides all the information of the *p* value **plus** it also takes into account sample size.
- Expressed in units of whatever the confidence interval applies to.

Bias

Bias is 'any process at any stage of inference which tends to produce results or conclusions that differ from the truth' (Sackett[3]).

Sources of bias in primary studies

- **Selection bias** – the subjects selected to be in the study (i.e. the sample population) may be different in some way from the population you aim to investigate.
- **Subject bias** – if the subject knows they are being observed or tested in some way they may behave differently to how they would normally.
- **Observer bias** – if the observer is aware of the aim of the study, the hypothesis being tested or whether the subject is in a treatment or control group, their assessment of the characteristics of interest may be biased. Sometimes this can be overcome by making sure the assessor is blind to allocation but this is not always possible.
- **Recall bias** – this may occur in retrospective studies, e.g. case-control studies when there is a difference in knowledge between subjects in the case and control groups leading to a biased recall. For example 'cases' may more readily recall exposure to a particular agent which may be associated with a disease than the 'controls'.

- **Information bias** – includes observer and recall bias.
- **Confounding bias** – occurs when a confounding factor is associated with both the suspected risk factor and the disorder.

Confounding variables/factors
- Should always be considered in interpreting results, especially non-randomised or observational studies.

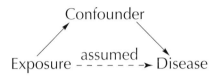

- These are associated with both the outcome of a study and the independent variables of interest (the exposure).
- Confounders have more influence upon outcome than the independent variables.

Type I error
- Occurs when the null hypothesis is rejected even though it is true.
- A statistical difference is found between two groups even though no true difference exists.
- Also called a **false positive** result.
- The probability of making a Type I error is equal to the p value and expressed as alpha (α – typically set at 0.05).
- Reasons for Type I errors are bias and confounding.

Type II error
- Occurs when the null hypothesis is accepted whereas the null hypothesis is in fact false.
- The study failed to detect a true difference between groups.
- A **false negative** result.
- Represented by beta (β – typically set at 0.2).
- Related to the **power** of the study.

Power
- Probability of rejecting the null hypothesis when a true difference exists.

- Represented by $(1-\beta) = 0.8$ or 80% power – the level normally seen as acceptable.
- Complex relationship dependent upon:
  - sample size
  - size of effect
  - reliability of measures
  - adopted significance level
- Therefore adequate power is achieved by:
  - large sample size
  - large effect sizes
  - high reliability
  - 0.05 significance level

Screening and diagnosis

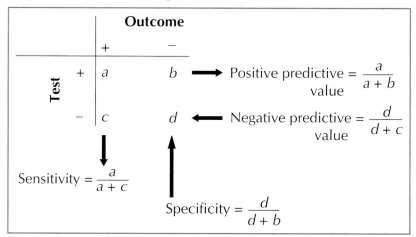

Sensitivity
- Ability to diagnose disease when present.
- **Probability of diagnosing disease when present.**
- Those who have the outcome/disease that are correctly identified as positive by the test.

Specificity
- Ability to identify absence of disease when disease is not present.
- **Probability of not diagnosing the disease when absent.**

- Those who do not have outcome/disease that are correctly identified as negative by the test.

Positive predictive value (PPV)

- The proportion of individuals who are identified as positive on the test **who are in fact** positive (have the disease/outcome).

Negative predictive value (NPV)

- The proportion of individuals identified as negative by the test **who are in fact** negative (do not have the disease/outcome).

Likelihood ratio for a positive result

- $\dfrac{\text{sensitivity}}{(1 - \text{specificity})}$ (true positives)
  (false positives)

- The likelihood that a positive test result will be observed in a patient as opposed to one without the disorder.
- Many reports of diagnostic tests provide multilevel likelihood ratios as measures of their accuracy.

Likelihood ratio for a negative result

- $\dfrac{(1 - \text{sensitivity})}{\text{specificity}}$ (false negatives)
  (true negatives)

Pre-test odds

- $\dfrac{\text{prevalence}}{(1 - \text{prevalence})} = \dfrac{\dfrac{(a + c)}{(a + b + c + d)}}{1 - \dfrac{(a + c)}{(a + b + c + d)}}$

Post-test odds

- Pre-test odds × likelihood ratio.

Post-test probability

- $\dfrac{\text{post-test odds}}{(\text{post-test odds} + 1)}$ (converts odds to risk)

Pre-test probability

- Same as prevalence $= \dfrac{(a + c)}{(a + b + c + d)}$

Key point

- Remember risk (probability) $= \dfrac{\text{odds}}{(1 + \text{odds})}$ and odds $= \dfrac{\text{risk}}{(1 - \text{risk})}$

Nomogram

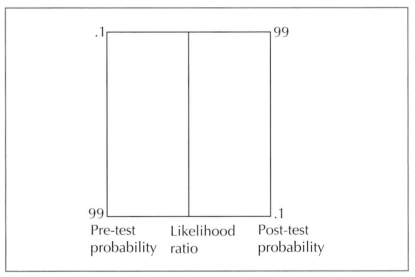

Fig. 6.1 A likelihood ratio nomogram. Adapted from Fagan,[4] as used in Sackett et al.[5]

A nomogram can be used to interpret diagnostic test results, to help you decide whether a diagnostic test produces important changes from pre-test to post-test probabilities.

Reliability

- Relates to the level of agreement between repeated measurements.
- Implies diagnostic consistency.

Measures of reliability

- **Inter-rater** – the level of agreement between assessments of the same material made by two or more assessors at roughly the same time.
- **Intra-rater** – the level of agreement between assessments of the same material made by the same assessor at two or more different times (with videoed or tape recorded material).
- **Test–re-test** – the level of agreement or correlation between repeat administration of the test under similar circumstances.
- **Alternative forms** – two forms of the same test are created and administered at the same time or consecutively.
- **Split half** – the test or measurement is administered, split in half, then the scores on one half are correlated with the other half.
- Statistical tests of reliability:
  - percentage agreement
  - product moment correlation coefficient
  - kappa statistic
  - intra-class correlation coefficient

Validity

- Term used to determine whether a particular test measures what it aims to measure. The extent to which it corresponds to a 'gold standard' or how well diagnoses compare to external validators (e.g. concurrent symptoms, cause of illness, diagnostic stability, biological markers, familial pattern, response to treatment).
- Validity is dependent on reliability.

Types of validity

- **Face validity** – on the surface does the test appear to be measuring what you are trying to measure? Not strictly a true type of validity.
- **Content validity** – similar concept but less superficial. Do the specific measurements aimed for by the

instrument assess the content of the measurement in question?

- **Predictive (prognostic) validity** – the extent of agreement between the test and a test in the future or predicted outcome.
- **Concurrent validity** – how does the test compare to already existing established tests or some sort of external validator?
- **Criterion validity** – predictive and concurrent validity are sometimes referred to together as criterion validity.
- **Incremental validity** – is the test/measure superior to other measures in approaching true validity?
- **Cross validity** – after a test has been criterion validated on one sample does it maintain criterion validity when applied to another sample?
- **Convergent validity** – do different measures of the same construct produce the same outcome and are they correlated?
- **Divergent validity** – does the test discriminate between other measures of unrelated constructs?
- **Construct validity** – constructs are abstract concepts and difficult to measure directly. Construct validity includes convergent and divergent validity and is connected with the underlying theory which is the basis of the test/instrument.

Randomised controlled trials (RCTs)

What is a randomised control trial?

- A trial in which subjects are randomly assigned to two or more groups (i.e. have an equal chance of being allocated to any group).
- The experimental group receives the intervention that is being tested.
- The comparison or control groups receive alternative treatments.
- The groups are followed up to see if any differences are evident, which can then be attributed to the new intervention.

CONSORT guidelines (Altman[6])

- All patients assessed for the trial should be accounted for plus the report should be accompanied by a guideline that explains what happened to all the patients involved in the trial.
- The randomisation procedure should be clearly specified.
- Inclusion plus exclusion criteria should be clearly stated.
- The method of blinding should be specified.
- There should be an **intention to treat** analysis.

Randomisation

- A procedure that ensures all subjects recruited to a trial have an equal chance of being allocated to the treatment or control groups.
- The purpose is to eliminate the **bias** which occurs when experimenters are allowed to influence subject allocation.
- The aim is to provide two or more identical groups of patients so that any differences observed can be attributed to the different treatments.
- Potentially **confounding** variables should be evenly distributed throughout the randomised groups.
- If confounders are known (e.g. age), sometimes stratification is used.
- The gold standard method of randomisation is the production of a **computer generated random number** at a **site distant from study** done by an **independent person** with good **concealment**.

Power calculation

- This is used to determine how many subjects are required for a clinical trial to have a good chance of detecting a clinically significant difference on a particular outcome variable – **if there is a difference**.

- $\dfrac{\text{Clinically significant difference}}{\text{sd}} \longrightarrow$ table of power for given number of subjects

80% power is the generally accepted cut-off $(1-\beta)$ (β = Type II error).

Intention to treat analysis

- Data on all randomised subjects are analysed within the groups to which they were assigned.
- Any other policy towards dropouts will involve subjective decisions, plus will create an opportunity for bias.
- Dropouts are an important group and therefore must be included. This group is relevant to clinical practice ('real life').

Informed consent

- The patient should understand the nature and purpose of the study and any risks and benefits of the intervention/treatment.
- The patient should understand that if they refuse to participate, normal treatment will not be affected.
- They should know that they can withdraw at any time without giving a reason and without affecting their treatment.
- They should know they have an equal chance of being allocated to control and treatment groups.
- The explanation should be given orally and in writing. They should have time to consider before deciding.
- A detailed discussion of research ethics is provided in Prothero,[7] and also at the Central Office for Research Ethics Committees (www.corec.org.uk).

Blinding

May mean:

- The patient is unaware whether they are in the treatment or control group.
- The therapist/investigator is unaware of group allocation.
- Both (**double blind**) – the strongest research design.

Common problems in RCTs

If you know a list of problems in all RCTs you can apply these to a specific paper in the exam:
- Failures of true randomisation.
- Inadequate concealment.
- Lack of blind treatment or outcome assessment.
- Ignoring missing data.
- Inappropriate and/or too many outcome measures.
- Patients likely to give informed consent and participate in the trial are often different from the 'average' patient. For example, in psychiatry, patients with more than one diagnosis or concurrent substance abuse are often excluded from RCTs.
- The development of **pragmatic trials** aims to overcome some of these criticisms.

Experimental event rate (EER)
- The rate of a dichotomous outcome in the group receiving the new intervention.
- Event may be positive (e.g. recovery) or negative (e.g. dropouts/side effects, etc.).
- Can be expressed as % or fraction.

Control event rate (CER)
- The rate of dichotomous outcome in the group receiving control or standard intervention.

Relative risk reduction (RRR)
- The proportional reduction in event rates between the treatment groups:

$$\frac{CER - EER}{EER}$$

Absolute risk reduction (ARR)
- Absolute difference in event rates in exceptional and control groups.

$$EER - CER = ARR \text{ (expressed as \% or fraction).}$$

Number needed to treat (NNT)
- Clinically useful measure of a treatment's value.
- The number of people one needs to treat with a specific intervention to achieve one **additional** favourable outcome.
- Calculated by: $\dfrac{1}{ARR}$

Effect size
- Often reported in terms of sd units or odds ratio.
- $\dfrac{\text{Difference between two means}}{\text{Standard deviation}}$ (Cohen's d) (standardised difference)
- Numerically equivalent to z scores.

Case control and cohort studies

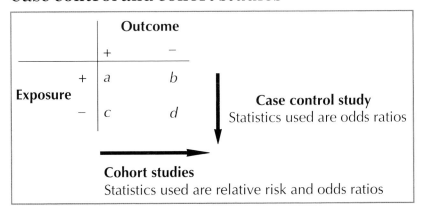

Case control study
- Usually retrospective but can also be prospective, cross-sectional and longitudinal.
- May be only way to investigate a **rare** disease/outcome.
- Controls should come from the same population as the cases but not have the disease.
- Can only demonstrate **association**, not causation.

Example:

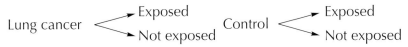

Cohort study
- Prospective.
- (Ideally) an **inception cohort** is followed up over time and outcome assessed.
- Can take years (e.g. decades).

Example:

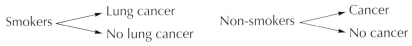

Probability

- The likelihood of any event occurring relative to (as a proportion of) the total number of possibilities. For example, in a drawer of red and green socks only, the probability of picking a green sock will be:

$$\frac{\text{no. of green socks}}{(\text{no. of green socks} + \text{no. of red socks})}$$

- Probability = risk.

Odds

- The odds of picking a green sock would be:

$$\frac{\text{no. of green socks}}{\text{no. of red socks}}$$

Converting risk to odds:

$$\text{Risk} = \frac{\text{odds}}{(1 + \text{odds})} \qquad \text{odds} = \frac{\text{risk}}{(1 - \text{risk})}$$

Odds ratio

- A measure of the strength of a treatment effect or an aetiological association, calculated by comparing outcome rates in exposed and non-exposed patients.
- The ratio of odds of an outcome in the experimental group, divided by the odds of an outcome in the other group.

$$\bullet \quad \frac{\text{Odds of exposure if have the disease/outcome}}{\text{Odds of exposure if don't have the disease/outcome}} = \frac{a/c}{b/d} = \frac{ad}{bc}$$

$$\bullet \quad \frac{\text{Odds of disease/outcome if exposed}}{\text{Odds of disease/outcome if not exposed}} = \frac{a/b}{c/d} = \frac{ad}{bc}$$

Relative risk

- The ratio of risk of outcome in one experimental group divided by risk of outcome in the other group.

$$\bullet \quad \frac{\text{Incidence in those exposed}}{\text{Incidence in those not exposed}} = \frac{a/a + b}{c/c + d} = \frac{a\,(c + d)}{c\,(a + b)}$$

Why calculate the odds ratio?

- You cannot calculate relative risk in case-control studies because you have no information about incidence.
- But if the disease is rare and the incidence is small, the odds ratio approximates to relative risk. Therefore in these cases it is useful to calculate the odds ratio.
- Statistically this is because:

$$RR = \frac{a\,(c+d)}{c\,(a+b)} \quad \longrightarrow \quad \approx \frac{ad}{bc}$$

If disease is rare a and c are relatively small numbers.

Systematic reviews and meta-analysis

Systematic reviews

- Pre-specify types of article to be included and excluded.
- Use specific search strategies to identify relevant articles.
- Cite all identified articles.
- Have some system for measuring quality of different studies.
- A detailed description of the process of carrying out a systematic review is given in Glanville.[8]

Meta-analysis

- Individual trials often have different or conflicting results.
- 'Rate counting' techniques do not assess quality and have lower power.
- Meta-analyses derive a quantitative summary of effect size by statistically combining effect sizes weighted by study size/quality.
- They can be non-systematic.
- They cannot combine non-randomised trials with RCTs.
- They are sensitive to:
  - **publication** bias
  - **location** bias
  - **inclusion** bias[9]

- They are influenced by the quality of the original trials.
- They are unreliable if event rates are low and number of studies small.
- They may give unreliable precision in observation studies.
- They may disagree with results from the largest RCT.

Reporting meta-analyses

When a number of studies have all examined the same outcome, their data can be combined. It is bad science to calculate a simple average as this would imply every study is as well-designed and completed as each other. In reality some studies are better carried through than others and are more likely to provide an accurate finding. More weight is therefore given to the 'best' and most informative studies. The 'best' studies usually have larger samples, are well-designed and show low homogeneity (see later). Results of the combination of studies and the different weighting allocated to studies is most commonly reported using Forest Plots. This is a graphical display which summarises key data both for individual studies and the combined totals. A vertical central line represents zero effect and is drawn at 1 (i.e. no difference). Boxes (reflecting the weighting allocated to the individual study) and horizontal lines (representing the confidence interval) summarise each study. A diamond shape summarises the total combined effect for all studies. An example of the structure of a Forest Plot is given below. Use the frequent examples in the *British Medical Journal* and other journals to practise the interpretation of these plots.

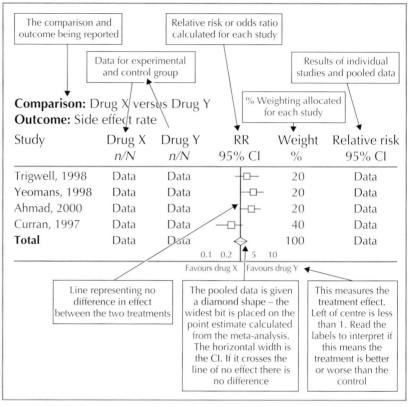

A Test for heterogeneity is included as a Chi square.

Finally a *Z* test summarising the overall effect is stated together with a *p* value to reflect the overall effect.

Publication bias

- The tendency for researchers to only write up and submit research with a positive result.
- Tendency for journals to accept and publish articles with a positive result.
- More evident in observational and intervention studies.
- Often associated with other types of bias; it is important to evaluate and control for this bias.

Location bias

- Language (e.g. omit foreign language journals in a systematic review).
- Database (only examine certain abstracting databases such as Medline and omit a significant part of the relevant literature as a result).
- Citation (mention only studies identified by others).
- Multiple publication (the same data presented as if it represents more than one study).

Inclusion bias

- Bias may arise in establishing the inclusion criteria for a meta-analysis.
- If the inclusion criteria are developed by an investigator familiar with the field of study the criteria may be influenced by the knowledge of the results of the potential studies.[9]

Heterogeneity

- Heterogeneity is a systematic difference in the effects in different studies beyond that expected by chance.
- Substantial heterogeneity between studies can bias the summary effect and may reflect important methodological differences and/or mean there are different sub-groups of patients, therefore it is important to identify this bias.
- Methods of testing heterogeneity:
    - 'eyeball' **funnel plot**
    - calculate **Q statistic**
    - **Galbraith plot** (identifies which studies contribute most to heterogeneity)

Summary estimates and calculation

- Meta-analysis calculates **summary effect size** (odds ratio) by taking the mean of all the individual study effect sizes 'weighted' by the individual study size.
- Weighting is done according to standard error either by:
    - **fixed effects modelling**: assumes each study is an estimate of a single underlying effect (i.e. favours large studies).

– **random effects modelling**: assumes all studies included are a true random sample of all studies.

Other types of studies to know about

- Surveys.
- Single case studies.
- Qualitative studies.
- Economic analysis.

Acknowledgements
We wish to thank Helen Prince for her helpful comments on this chapter.

Key points

- Read key texts concerning critical appraisal and research methodology (e.g. Crombie,[1] Lawrie et al,[2] Sackett et al[5]).
- Statistical and research definitions are often defined in a number of books. Use the current chapter to help identify areas that you should both understand and be able to define.
- Learning the definitions by rote is not enough. You must attempt to **understand the concepts** involved.
- Read about the different definitions and terms using different sources and practise applying them to the papers that you read in order to reinforce your learning.

REFERENCES

1. Crombie IK (1996) *The Pocket Guide to Critical Appraisal*. BMJ Books: London.

2. Lawrie S, McIntosh A, Rao A (2000) *Critical Appraisal for Psychiatry*. Churchill Livingstone: London.

3. Sackett DL (1979) Bias in analytic research. *Journal of Chronic Disease* 32: 51–63. Taken from: Johnstone EC, Freeman CPL, Zealley AK (1990) *Companion to Psychiatric Studies*, Sixth Edition. Churchill Livingstone: London.

4. Fagan TJ (1975) Nomogram from Bayes's theorem (c). *New England Journal of Medicine* 293: 257.

5. Sackett DL, Scott W, Richardson MD, Rosenberg W, Haynes RB (1996) *Evidence Based Medicine*. Churchill Livingstone: London.

6. Altman AG (1996) Better reporting of randomised controlled trials: the CONSORT statement. *British Medical Journal* 313: 570–571.

7. Prothero A (1999) Ethical issues in research. In: Curran S, Williams CJ (1999) *A Practical Guide to Clinical Research in Psychiatry*. Butterworth Heinemann: Oxford.

8. Glanville J (1999) Carrying out the literature search. In: Curran S, Williams CJ (1999) *A Practical Guide to Clinical Research in Psychiatry*. Butterworth Heinemann: Oxford.

9. Egger M, Davey Smith G (1990) Meta-analysis bias in location and selection of studies. *British Medical Journal* 316: 61–66.

OTHER USEFUL REFERENCES

• Bowers D (2002) *Medical Statistics from Scratch*. Wiley & Sons: Chichester.

• Puri BK, Tyrer PJ (1998) *Sciences Basic to Psychiatry*. Churchill Livingstone: Edinburgh.

• Puri B, Hall AD (2004) *Revision Notes in Psychiatry*, 2nd Edition. Arnold: London.

Essay technique

David Yeomans

The Part II exam includes an essay paper which lasts 90 minutes. Candidates are required to answer one from three questions. All three questions in the paper encompass aspects of general adult psychiatry and one or more of the different psychiatric specialties.

Possible essay topics

General psychiatry questions may cover a surprising range of topics:

- Clinical
- Epidemiology
- Diagnostic systems
- Need for psychiatric services/setting up services
- Rehabilitation
- Transcultural psychiatry
- Hospital liaison
- Neuropsychiatry
- HIV
- Medicine relevant to psychiatry
- Research

Psychiatric specialties may include topics such as:
- Child and adolescent
- Forensic
- Learning disability
- Psychiatry of old age
- Psychotherapy

Preparation

When you draw up your revision timetable be sure to set aside regular time to practise essays. Writing is physically tiring and is a skill that you may not have practised for several years. By the end of your revision you should have written 10–20 essay plans and at least two full length pieces.

Reading is your major source of factual information. You cannot read everything, so be selective:

- Review articles in major journals (e.g. *British Journal of Psychiatry*) and review journals (e.g. *Current Opinion, Psychiatry and Advances in Psychiatric Practice*) are useful. Read the exam syllabus (from Royal College of Psychiatrists) to see which areas you need to know and which you don't. Send off for past papers and obtain the most recent exam papers from colleagues who have recently taken the exam. Lists of recent exam questions are commonly reproduced on examination revision sites on the internet.
- Work out what major topics you wish to cover. Many candidates find it useful to produce a collection of 'essay plans'. If you prepare 15–20 topics, some of them may be included in the actual exam.

Essay spotting

There are several assumptions underlying the technique of essay spotting:

- Certain topics are important and these tend to be repeated.
- If such a topic has not come up recently then the chances of it appearing as a question in the next exam may be increased.
- Currently topical issues may be set on the essay paper (e.g. nationwide changes in service provision, Mental Health Act, prominent review articles). Look at the editorials and reviews that have appeared in the last 12 months of the *Psychiatric Bulletin* and the *British Journal of Psychiatry*.

The choice of essays on the paper is very limited (one from three). As a result, some candidates may immediately discount the possibility of being able to answer **any** of the questions at all. If you concentrate on using effective essay technique during your preparation and on the day of the exam, however, you will be able to make a good attempt at writing the essay required. On first seeing the paper, do not automatically discount **any** of the questions. **Stop and think** how you might answer each question before making your choice.

The techniques outlined in this chapter can put you at an advantage over other candidates who will not have practised these techniques, let alone written an essay for many years.

Structuring an essay

What is an essay? It is a long written piece held together by a **structure** and contains **arguments** supported by **information**. A common structure for an essay is an **introduction**, then the **arguments**, followed by your **conclusion**. This basic structure may need to be modified depending on how the essay question is asked. A very open question such as 'Describe the uses of medical audit' requires you to define the structure yourself. A question such as 'Discuss the effects of antidepressants on the course and outcome of anxiety disorders' is more clearly defined, but you must still impose some structure on your answer. This can be done using the techniques described below.

- Spend a few minutes before you start writing to prepare an **essay plan**. Write out your essay structure at the beginning of the essay and label it as the essay outline. You can then refer back to it as you write in order to maintain the structure and keep track of the remaining time. Cross out those areas you have covered so that you can see how the essay is progressing. Take time to review the content intermittently in case any fresh ideas come to mind.
- Six useful questions are: **Who? What? Why? Where? When? How?** When tackling the essay, ask yourself these questions to help produce a critical discussion.

Think about what terms the question uses. **What** is medical audit? **Who** is interested in audit? **Why** should doctors get involved? **How** is anxiety defined? **How many** different antidepressants are there? **What** is outcome? **How** is it measured?

- **Helicoptering**. A helicopter can hover miles up in the sky to obtain a broad view of the situation. It can descend to various points in that landscape to see more details. You can do this in an essay by alternating between a general overview and more focused and detailed argument.

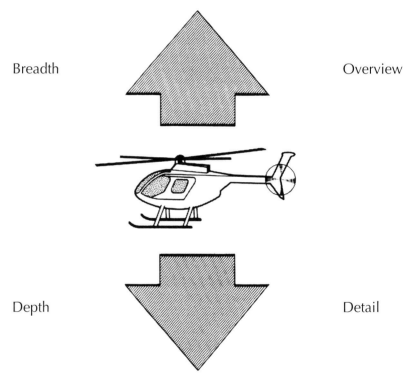

Breadth   Overview

Depth   Detail

Fig 7.1 Helicoptering.

Expansion techniques

Before setting pen to paper expand the question to its limits by considering all the subject areas you can include. Helpful sub-headings to expand the scope of your thinking (and hence your essay) include:

- Biological, psychological and social aspects.
- Acute, intermediate and long term.
- Male and female differences.
- Age differences.
- Cultural differences.
- Approaching the question from the point of view of different sub-specialties (such as child psychiatry, psychiatry of the elderly, liaison psychiatry, etc.).
- 'Non-medical' factors such as the impact on carers, media influences, voluntary sector supports, politics and finance.
- Past, present and future implications.

The Royal College website provides some helpful suggestions on the process of writing the essay – especially that "the essay paper requires candidates **to integrate knowledge** rather than to repeat facts, **to synthesise diverse information**, and **to develop a reasoned argument**. Candidates are expected **to communicate their views succinctly** and clearly and **to demonstrate knowledge** of relevant literature". You should address these items in bold as you write the essay.

Worked example 1

Candidates on our *MRCPsych Part II Examination Techniques* course were asked to use the above techniques to create essay plans. Although no one felt prepared for the task, one group produced the following essay structure within 10 minutes.

Question
Discuss medical classification and how it has been applied in psychiatry.

Answer
INTRODUCTION: Why is classification necessary?

- Communication.
- Universal use.
- Predict prognosis.
- It aids research so that different researchers can study similar patients.
- Implications for treatment.

CLASSIFICATION METHODS
- Syndromal: grouping of symptoms and signs.
- Aetiology: infective, trauma, genetic, etc.
- Course: acute, chronic or remitting.
- Outcome.
- Multi-axial definitions (or a combined biopsychosocial model).

APPLICATION OF CLASSIFICATION MODELS IN PSYCHIATRY
- The current systems: ICD, DSM.
- Historical perspective: e.g. Kraepelin.

PROBLEMS AND CHALLENGES IN CLASSIFICATION
- Lack of reliability in rating.
- Lack of construct validity (e.g. schizophrenia – key papers).
- Results of statistical analyses (e.g. cluster and factor analysis) fails to support many diagnostic constructs.
- Problems result from labelling/stigma – key papers.
- Lack of success, lack of clear aetiologies and the limitations of syndromal classification.
- Outcome predictions are actually quite poor.

CONCLUSIONS
- Slow but steady progress is being made.
- More consensus than before.
- Future hope to include more aetiological and pathological data with multi-axial descriptions taken into account.
- Problem and symptom focused assessments may show more benefits in future.

This essay structure demonstrates some of the techniques described above. First of all, you **must read the question in full**. A simple approach with an introduction, arguments, and conclusion is used. There is a clear structure. The candidates in this case defined **what** classification is and **why** it is used. They focused down from the two broad questions on classification and application and split each up into several headings. For some of the headings they focused down further to give detailed examples which illustrate the benefits and pitfalls of using diagnostic systems. They then 'helicoptered' up again to allow a wider discussion of the arguments. The essay structure is **critical** and asks **how successful** classification is in psychiatry. The content and structure clearly considers different aspects of the answer and develops these logically. It looks to **what** the future may hold and expands the question a little beyond what was asked. Perhaps it could have included some consideration of cultural differences and similarities. You may already have different ideas of how you would answer this question. Why not try them out now?

Worked example 2

Question
How can exploratory psychotherapy lead to a worsening of a patient's condition? What can be done to reduce this?
Think for a few minutes before you read the possible answer below.

Answer
INTRODUCTION
Definitions:
(a) **Exploratory psychotherapy:** dynamic psychotherapy; types/methods; individual/group/family; in children and adults.
(b) **Worsening:**
   (i)   In therapy: transference/counter-transference issues; risks of dependency. Risks of

> reawakening upsetting memories and worsening distress.
> **(ii)** Out of therapy: acting out; also to consider problems in work or with their family.
> **(iii)** General: risks of parasuicide/self-harm; anxiety or depression.
> **(iii)** Risks directly related to therapy: e.g. abusive or controlling therapist, or an unqualified psychotherapist who has not undergone a professional training and who is unsupervised.
>
> ### ARGUMENTS
> These went on to discuss the above ideas, and particularly to discuss the 'worsening' in terms of overall outcome.
>
> ### WHAT CAN BE DONE TO PREVENT WORSENING?
> - Patient selection including liaison with referrers.
> - Training and supervision of psychotherapists. Statutory regulations of psychotherapists – possibly through the Health Professions Council (HPC).
> - Conjoint work and treatment (e.g. additional medication from general practitioners).
> - The importance of clear communication and continuity of treatment.
> - Monitor the mental state closely.
> - Assess defence mechanisms for potential vulnerability to psychological treatment approaches.
> - Pay attention to transference and counter-transference issues and difficulties.
> - Give adequate preparation for times of absence by the therapist.
> - Consider the frequency of sessions and the risks of dependency occurring.

The candidates' reaction to this essay title was interesting. Initially they felt great pessimism when given this question to attempt. They said that they would never have chosen this topic in an exam, and believed that they would answer it very badly because they did not have any specialised expertise in this field. None expected to produce such an extensive outline until they applied the techniques taught above. They were surprised to find out exactly how much they really knew. Had this been the only question they could remotely hope to answer, this technique-based approach would have given them a much better chance of success.

Self-test followed by worked example 3

Now write an essay plan and a full essay under exam conditions (90 minutes solid, no textbooks). The title of your essay is "***Discuss ways of improving physical health in schizophrenia***".

A guide to the technique and a full essay written by the author under exam conditions is given below. Do your essay before reading the example. (The author has an unfair advantage because he has an interest in the area.) Use the techniques above to brainstorm the issues in this question, then choose an essay plan structure before writing the full essay. Write all your notes and plan in the essay paper but clearly marked as your 'working'.

---

1) Planning your answer

a) Brainstorm the issues

Who	should do what? – refer to NICE, GP contact
What	works? – weight management, smoking cessation
Why	bother? – because of high mortality rates
Where	should patients go for help? – primary versus secondary care
When	to intervene? – during clinics, in special meetings
How	do psychiatrists learn the skills to help, get the resources?

---

b) Overview

High mortality rates, patchy services, equality of access, social exclusion, public policy.

Detail: e.g. Specific difficulties interpreting a specialised test such as serum prolactin concentration.

c) Expand the scope

Biopsychosocial	motivation to change lifestyle, cultural pressures, genetics
Acute/long term	long time to see weight reduction benefits so no immediate reinforcement
Male/female	views on weight/attractiveness/fitness
Age	increases risk of diabetes
Culture	growing concern over obesity
Political	government health departments have an increased focus/costs MI, CVA diabetes, etc.
Subspecialties	primary or secondary care input
Non-medical	drug companies interests
Past/present/future	professional development need

d) Ask yourself, what have I read or heard about?

- NICE guidance on schizophrenia has a section on physical health.
- Rethink did a survey including opinions on physical health.
- GPs have a new contract with points for physical health monitoring in severe mental illness.
- Drug companies tell me about side effects.
- Our depot clinic weighs people and runs a diet group.

Based on these thoughts, impose a structure on these ideas to produce an essay plan.

2) Create an essay plan

Background
The research evidence and public policy that defines the issues and sets the scene for action to improve physical health in schizophrenia.

Improving physical health : the actions that can be taken including
Lifestyle assessment, physical examination and screening tests, side effect measurement, health promotion, lifestyle change, treatment review, health improvement programmes.

Continuing professional development
The requirements on staff to upgrade their skills to meet the challenge of physical health.

Summary
A short paragraph outlining the whole essay in brief.

Finally, based on this plan, write out your essay in full.

3) Full essay example
Discuss ways of improving physical health in schizophrenia

Introduction and background
Physical health is becoming a bigger issue in schizophrenia because there is a growing evidence base for higher than average physical morbidity and mortality in severe mental illness (Harris and Barraclough, 1998). GPs and psychiatrists are being asked to routinely assess and treat physical health problems. GPs get points for running severe mental illness registers and performing physical health checks on all patients with severe mental illness. Psychiatrists are required by NICE guidelines to monitor physical health for patients with schizophrenia who cannot access primary care.

Burns and Cohen (1998) found that providing equal access to primary care was a challenge for patients with severe mental illness. Harris and Barraclough (1998) demonstrated that patients with schizophrenia have higher than average standardised mortality rates from natural causes, especially from respiratory disease. Brown et al (1999) found that schizophrenic patients had unhealthy lifestyles with high fat, low fibre diets and high rates of smoking. Ryan et al (2003) have found a higher incidence of impaired glucose tolerance in drug-naïve, first episode schizophrenics.

It is difficult to encourage equal access to primary care but the needs of patients with schizophrenia are higher than average. People with schizophrenia are at higher risk of developing physical ill health; they engage in activities with high risks for physical ill health such as smoking (Kelly, Nithsdale studies) and they have poorer health outcomes including higher mortality.

Other causes of physical ill health in schizophrenia include side-effects of treatment.

Antipsychotic medications can lead to increased appetite, weight gain, hyperprolactinaemia, sexual impairment, parkinsonism, dyskinesias, sedation, as well as cognitive and emotional adverse effects. It is not clear whether some antipsychotics are worse than others, although there may be class differences between typical and atypical antipsychotics. Issues around side effects on physical health have a significant influence on which drugs are prescribed. Several drug companies are developing information resources and services in the area of physical health in severe mental illness.

Improving physical health

There are several ways to improve health. There are many health promotion activities for the general population and we should aim to provide equal access to those with schizophrenia. People with schizophrenia are often poor, live alone, are unemployed and have little support from others.

They visit their GPs often but get less health promotion there than average (Burns and Cohen, 1998). Physical health may be improved by better access to existing health promotion. This can be tackled by mental health care staff promoting physical health in the course of their mental health jobs. Rethink reported that regular physical health check-ups feature in the top three priorities for improving services in almost a third of their 3033 survey respondents ("Just one percent", 2003). Clinicians can discuss lifestyle. Lifestyle change, by the patient, is probably the most potent route for improving physical health. The Diabetes Prevention Research Group (*New England Journal of Medicine*, 2002) found that lifestyle intervention was more effective than metformin in reducing the cumulative incidence of diabetes in high risk persons. Clinicians can provide information on smoking, alcohol and drug use and provide access to services that help quit using high risk substances. Sexual health can be addressed in the same way. Clinicians should ask directly about sexual dysfunction and equip themselves with the skills to address sexual health problems through continuing professional development. It is not too difficult to provide clinics with weighing scales, and a scale for height measurement. This allows the measurement of body mass index (weight in kg/height in m^2). We would probably find over 75% of our patients were overweight and thus at increased risk of cardiovascular disease and diabetes. Adding blood pressure measurement and some blood screens such as FBC, LFTs, U&Es, TFTs, random glucose and prolactin would help detect a range of physical health problems. It would be ideal to perform baseline screens before starting treatment with antipsychotics, so that other causes of abnormal results could be assessed. Abnormally high prolactin levels are common with antipsychotics, but also occur with pituitary tumours. A baseline normal prolactin followed by a high prolactin after medication would indicate a tumour was unlikely. Without a baseline it is hard to tell without stopping medication and repeating the prolactin test.

In addition to health discussions, lifestyle assessment and health screening, we can provide direct services or links to primary care and voluntary sector provision. There is a national smoking cessation programme, free nicotine substitutes and local programmes. GPs can prescribe exercise – with, for example, free access to gyms paid for by the NHS. Established businesses offer weight reduction programmes (e.g. weight watchers) and gym facilities. Many people want to use normal services to address problems of weight. However, for the reasons given earlier, many people with schizophrenia cannot use these services. Being poor, paranoid and unmotivated is not conducive to getting out and getting healthier. People with schizophrenia may attend clinics and day centres and have contact with staff in community teams, depot clinics and day hospitals. In these settings it is possible to set up groups to encourage reflection on physical health, and to encourage lifestyle change, for example, by introducing a healthy cooking or aerobics slot. By building on existing engagement with staff, people can be encouraged to take part in group activities, such as walking, bowling, cooking, shopping, cycling and swimming. With appropriate help from support workers, people can use the local facilities available to all. Direct service provision is likely to be a long-term intervention. Research shows that weight loss is possible and persistent work over long periods increases benefit (Pendlebury).

Doctors have a big role to play in minimising physical harm from medication. One way to do this is to systematically enquire about side effects. Large screening questionnaires exist, like the LUNSERS developed in Liverpool (Bentall, Day et al), although brief systematic questioning could quickly explore the main areas of sexual dysfunction, sedation, weight gain, neuromuscular disorders and anti-cholinergic effects. Having found problems we need to decide on appropriate remedies, after an informed discussion of the pros and cons of treatment change. If major changes are needed then a crisis plan and advance plan can be set up with users, carers, staff and mediators if available.

Continuing professional development

Some clinicians will have understandable concerns about their skills in the area of physical health. These can be improved by learning from GPs, physicians, pharmacists and other colleagues in the course of daily working. Refreshing your knowledge from reading updates (e.g. in the *British Medical Journal*) can be helpful. Special courses in psychopharmacology exist and would improve confidence in pharmacotherapy. It is also instructive to keep a record of how patients respond to changes in lifestyle and treatment. Computer databases and spreadsheets allow records to be reviewed to see if interventions are working. This feeds into clinical governance mechanisms.

Summary

People with schizophrenia are at greater than average risk of physical health problems. Health staff can help by deciding it is within their role to offer information on lifestyles and physical illness. Further, we can routinely screen for health problems in high risk groups (such as psychosis) and offer treatment directly, or from colleagues. We can encourage people to take up healthier lifestyles. We can try to reduce side effects of treatment. In doing these things we are likely to help improve the physical health of people with schizophrenia. If we collect data on the outcomes of these interventions we will see just how effective we can be. This is a long term issue that needs careful monitoring. Specific resources would make it easier to implement. These are available in primary care but need further attention in secondary care.

The role of the examiner

The examiner has to mark multiple essays on the same question. Remember he or she may well be bored and would prefer to be doing something else. It is your task to present them with a clearly legible, well written, structured essay that stands out from all the others.

What to do

The instructions on the exam paper state:

> The answers should be written in *essay form*; in addition, tables and/or diagrams may be used wherever these add to the clarity of the candidate's account. The candidate is expected to communicate clearly, present arguments coherently, evaluate evidence and make balanced judgements. The answers should refer to the basic scientific, as well as clinical, aspects of each topic. Extra marks will be given for appropriate and critical reference to the literature and research findings. **Illegibility will be penalised**.
>
> Source: Royal College of Psychiatrists Examination Paper, 1999. Royal College of Psychiatrists, Belgrave Square, London.

Candidates who do not take these instructions seriously, particularly regarding legibility of handwriting, will have much greater difficulty in passing the exam.

What <u>not</u> to do

Don't just state facts. Instead you must use your **judgement in evaluating the information** and **arguing** your case. Don't make things up. Don't waffle about irrelevancies. Do not write about a totally different question just because you have prepared an essay plan about it. You will get no marks unless you answer the question that is

---

Important guidelines

- Write legibly.
- Consider writing double-spaced. This makes your essay easier on the eye and simpler to mark.
- Break up the text with headings, lists, diagrams and tables where appropriate. (Take a look at your textbooks and see how they present information. Each chapter in the book is itself an essay.) The College guidelines clearly state that the **use of tables and/or diagrams may be appropriate**.
- Use colour (e.g. a red pen) to highlight important points or sub-headings using underlining.
- Provide references where possible (name and year if you can, if not, state what you can remember, e.g. "A paper published in the British Journal of Psychiatry last month showed . . .").
- Write naturally, but consider the following. Short sentences add impact. Long sentences with no punctuation such as commas that go on for line after line and talk about different subjects without so much as a pause between them do tend to confuse and the examiner does not want to re-read the essay 10 times to work out what you are trying to say. See?
- Show the examiners that you can order information, and make the presentation and structure clear by the use of sub-headings.
- Bullet points can be very effective in lists.

asked. Remember this point when you have 'spotted' a question. You need to tailor the prepared answer to the question on the exam paper. Do not be unbalanced in your arguments. Remember that your essay reveals things about you. Examiners may be concerned if, for example, you appear to have no consideration for patients' well being. Finally, remember that an essay requires a reasonably lengthy piece of writing – one page is not enough!

What are your blindspots?

When you write a practice essay, ask someone to comment critically about it. You may be unaware of habitual spelling or grammatical errors. You may not notice a tendency to leave words unfinished (one of the authors has this proble). Let someone else discover your blindspots, but be critical of **their** criticism. In the end you have to rely on your own style.

> ### Key points
> - Read the questions carefully and answer the question you have been asked.
> - Answers should be written in essay form. You should communicate clearly, present coherent arguments, evaluate evidence and produce balanced judgements.
> - Structure your answer clearly. Illegibility will be penalised.
> - Use helicoptering to produce a broad overview and then focus on specific areas.
> - Use questions such as **Why? What? Where? When? How?** Take on different perspectives (child, adult, old age, etc.) to keep your answer broad.
> - Use expansion techniques.
> - Gain extra points by using reference to the literature.

Preparing for the long case (individual patient assessment)

Christopher Williams

The long case clinical examination occurs in the Part II exam and consists of 60 minutes with a single patient and then 30 minutes with the examiners.

The general principles of doing well in the clinical exams are to organise your knowledge, making what you say:

- Clear
- Relevant
- Interesting

Remember:

- Clear communicators consistently do well.
- You are presenting **yourself**, not merely the case.
- It is not a test of detailed academic knowledge; this is covered in the written papers.
- You are also being asked to demonstrate your skills as a clinician.

You need to demonstrate to the examiners that you are a safe, sensible and competent clinician who could be trusted to look after their patients.

Preparation

The good news is that you know in advance what areas the examiners are interested in. You will be asked to present your case summary, present and justify your differential diagnosis and go on to discuss possible management plans. To prepare for this:

- Know what is expected of you. Read the Royal College guidelines concerning the exam; these tell you about the content and structure of the exam.
- Take opportunities to present cases (ward rounds, clinic, etc.).
- Practise presenting cases under exam conditions. For some of the mock cases, make sure that you are asked to interview the patient in front of the mock examiner. This is something that is rarely practised, but is important.
- Seek supervised training in interviewing skills. Watch yourself presenting on video. This is a very effective way to identify what areas you need to change.

Mock clinical exams

Make sure that you do mock clinical exams on each of the main areas of psychiatry. These are common problems seen in psychiatric practice, and hence are common in exams:

- Depressive disorder.
- Schizophrenia.
- Anxiety disorders.
- Obsessive-compulsive disorder.
- Alcohol abuse/dependence.
- Eating disorders.

If possible, do mock exams with a variety of **different examiners** who have different theoretical and clinical backgrounds. Do not just ask 'friendly' examiners who you know well. Seek out those with a range of examining styles. If there are any College examiners at the hospital where you work, you should try to carry out at least one exam with them as well. Be willing to accept their feedback and suggestions to change. Ultimately, however, you are seeking to develop a clinical interview and presentation style with which **you** are happy.

MOCK CLINICAL EXAM ASSESSMENT SHEET

Examiner: **Candidate:**

General: The ability to pick out the salient features of the case and present these clearly and coherently is stressed. The organisation of information is particularly important.

History taking: Is what is presented systematic and comprehensive with no omissions? Logically presented and structured?

Mental state examination: Systematic and comprehensive with no omissions?

Interview of the patient: Sensitive interview, good rapport, fluent interview style? Put patient at ease, good empathy? Good use of open then closed questions? Systematic and comprehensive with no omissions? The ability to firmly but politely control the interview without dominating, and at the same time cover the appropriate clinical questions quickly, clearly and efficiently should be assessed.

Physical assessment: Can recognise significant findings and identify their importance/relevance?

Overall impression/diagnosis of the case: Diagnostic skills, knowledge of aetiology including psychological aspects? Knowledge of diagnostic classification systems? Pay particular regard to social and psychological treatments, as well as purely physical approaches.

Presentation: Clear communicator and good delivery, articulate, clarity of presentation?

The assessment of **relevant physical factors** should be recognised in the mark. (7–10 minutes)

Interviewing the patient: Politeness and professional attitude? (5 minutes)

Overall mark: A general discussion with the candidate would probably be the most help rather than an overall statement of Pass or Fail.

Comments: Helpful ways to improve presentation and organisation of material?

(*Pass the MRCPsych*, Third Edition. Williams, Trigwell and Yeomans 2005)

When you do the practice exams, try to obtain **specific** feedback. This will help you identify your relatively stronger and weaker areas. An assessment sheet such as the one above may aid this and can be used by others (e.g. your peers in a study group) to rate your performance. You can also use it yourself if you are analysing your presentation on videotape.

Predicting and practising cases

Try and remember that the hospital where you sit the examination will tend to have the same types of patients that you see in your own clinical practice. The hospital has to provide approximately 20–30 patients for the exams and these are therefore likely to include both inpatients and outpatients. Think through in advance how you will assess, present and manage each of the following clinical cases. It is not necessary to carry out mock exams on each of these, but you should think each case through thoroughly. You may find it useful to either write down full assessment and management plans of a 'typical' case, or to test and be tested by peers who are also taking the exam.

> ### Write out full assessment and management plans for each of the following:
> - Major affective disorders.
> - Schizophrenia (and drug-induced psychosis).
> - Alcohol or substance abuse.
> - Anxiety disorders.
> - Obsessive-compulsive disorder.
> - Agoraphobia or other phobias.
> - Hypochondriasis/health anxiety and somatoform disorders.
> - Dementia (these patients will be accompanied by an informant).
> - Eating disorders.
> - Any area that the examining hospital specialises in.

> Do not attempt to visit or contact the clinical staff or wards of the hospital you will be examined at. This can lead to you being disqualified from the exam.
>
> It is possible that a patient with a learning disability or a child will take part in the exam. If so, they would always be accompanied by an informant.

Coming to the exam

Think:

- What impression do I want to give?
- What will I wear and how will I look?

How can I arrive on time?

It is surprising how often this causes problems. Expect the unexpected (traffic jams, rail strikes, losing your car keys, etc.). If you are late it will leave you feeling tense, pressured and unlikely to perform well. Consider staying overnight in a good hotel (not noisy). It is worth the money. A long drive with an early start on the day of the exam may be inadvisable, and being 'on-site' can make a big difference. If the hotel is poor or noisy, check out and move somewhere better. Passing the exam is worth more than the expense of an extra hotel bill.

The clinical assessment

Engaging the patient

- Introduce yourself to the patient.
- Explain that you need to take some notes to help you remember (especially important if the patient is experiencing paranoid beliefs).
- Apologise in advance for having to interrupt them; say why (it is an exam; time pressures, etc.).
- Be polite and professional.

Be organised as you take the history

Nothing creates an impression of disorganisation more than a flurry of paper during the presentation. This can be reduced by a few simple techniques:

- Write on only one side of the paper.
- Number the sheets.
- Organise your information clearly as you take the history.
- Use clear headings (personal history, family history, etc.).
- Consider writing the headings down at the start of the exam. This can help you pace your history taking, and also prevents you forgetting to ask about any central and important areas.

It is not the place here to go through in detail how to take a psychiatric history. This is described in all basic psychiatric textbooks. A good description is in *The Oxford Textbook of Psychiatry*.[1] We suggest that you read the chapters on the psychiatric history and mental state in detail and repeatedly practise areas such as testing the cognitive state.

- **Maintain momentum**. You cannot afford to run out of time.
- **Leave gaps** between each area on your history sheets. You are likely to forget some questions and this allows you to fit in later infor-

---

Presentation

While presenting the patient use a style most examiners will recognise. For example:

- Presenting complaint/history of presenting complaint.
- Personal history.
- Premorbid personality.
- Family history.
- Social history.
- Forensic history.
- Past medical history.
- Past psychiatric history (always including post-partum problems and deliberate self-harm).

- Drugs/allergies to drugs (do not forget depots or current ECT).
- Full mental state examination.
- Physical examination.

Always mention the presence or absence of suicidal ideas and behaviour.

mation without creating an unreadable mass of extra notes scribbled in margins.

- You can always ask the patient what diagnosis they have been given, and also what treatments or investigations they have had. This can offer very useful clues.
- Aim to finish in 45 minutes leaving you 15 minutes to gather your thoughts and plan your presentation. Ask the patient to stay while you review your notes and check what you have forgotten or need to clarify.
- Consider using a red pen or a highlighter to mark important key areas that you will later read out in the presentation.
- Thank the patient and mention that you will be asked to interview them again in front of the examiners.

An appropriate (often brief) physical examination should always be carried out and included in your presentation. This could include:

- Pulse.
- Blood pressure.
- Evidence of autonomic over-arousal (e.g. sweating, pallor, tremor).
- Stigmata of thyroid or liver disease.
- Evidence of previous injury (self-cutting, etc.).
- Anything else that is clearly relevant (e.g. they use a wheelchair).

Sometimes, patients may seem very complex. You can still pass by using a systematic approach to effective clinical assessment and presentation.

Clustering questions

A very important technique to learn is that of **clustering questions together**. In psychiatry, diagnoses are largely made by observing if particular symptoms aggregate together in patterns that are felt to represent specific disorders or syndromes. Most examiners have a model in their minds of the cluster of symptoms that make up each diagnosis (such as 'depressive disorder'). These clusters have been formalised in the various diagnostic systems such as ICD 10 and DSM IV. How then is this relevant to the exam situation?

Examiners do not have very much information about the patient you have seen. All they know is a basic written summary from the team looking after them. What you need to do is to **paint a picture** of the patient for them. In order to present this clearly to the examiners, it is vital to **cluster** symptoms together logically while taking the history, and therefore while presenting. This is the key to a good presentation. When, for example, you mention depressed mood the examiners will want to know if the patient fits their own (or the ICD) model of depression. They will therefore expect a description of not only how depressed the mood is, the presence of anhedonia, mood reactivity, etc., but also whether there is any evidence of 'biological' symptoms of depression, and to what extent the depression has affected the person's life.

Thus, if you are asking about depression **ask about all these areas at one time** so that your history contains a clear focused summary. Write the symptoms down on one part of the paper so that they are presented (clustered) clearly on your sheets, and hence when you present. Don't allow yourself to be distracted by the patient when taking the history. In some cases you may have to come back to clarify things later, but do this all on the same sheet of paper so that everything you have found out about a particular problem area is found together in that one spot. This will help you give a clear presentation.

Two typical 'clusters' of questions covering depression and anxiety are presented below. Each of these has a similar structure. Try to create your own individualised clusters which you will be able to remember easily. Practise these until you can go through them quickly and reliably.

Clustering symptoms of depression: a five areas CBT-style assessment[2]

1. The situation, relationship and practical problems faced.
2. **Altered thinking:** hopelessness, negative view of self/situation/future, suicidal ideas, etc.
3. **Altered feelings:** severity/reactivity/anhedonia, etc.
4. **Altered physical/biological symptoms:** diurnal variation of mood, poor appetite, weight loss, etc.
5. **The altered behaviour/activity levels:**
   - What have you stopped doing since becoming depressed?
   - What are you doing differently because of these problems?
   - How has it affected you, your family and work?

Clustering symptoms of anxiety: a five areas CBT-style assessment[2]

1. The situation, relationship and practical problems faced.
2. **Altered thinking:** catastrophic thinking, jumping to the worst conclusion, worry, etc.
3. **Altered feelings:** how severe is the anxiety? Is it generalised or focused as a phobic state? Does the anxiety ever rise to a crescendo and cause panic attacks?
4. **Altered physical/biological symptoms:** is there evidence of marked somatic anxiety? It can be helpful to cluster the questions by asking about evidence of sympathetic and/or parasympathetic symptoms, and also for any symptoms caused by hyperventilation:

Sympathetic nervous system:
- Rapid heart
- Palpitations
- Tremor
- Sweating
- Flushing

Parasympathetic nervous system:
- Nausea
- Vomiting
- Loose motions/diarrhoea
- Frequency of urine

Hyperventilation:
- Dizzy
- Blurred vision
- Depersonalisation/derealisation
- Sweating
- Dry mouth
- Chest pain
- Subjective shortness of breath

5. **Altered behaviour/activity:**
- What have you reduced or stopped doing because of your problems (reduced activity or avoidance)?
- What are you doing differently because of these problems (?unhelpful behaviours such as drinking excessively)?

Is there any evidence of **avoidance**? This has important implications for treatment.

Create your own **symptom-cluster checklists** asking about paranoid ideas/schizophrenia, alcoholism/substance misuse, eating disorders, obsessive-compulsive disorder, etc. You will find that the skills learned in doing this will also be useful for the time when you have to interview the patient in front of the examiners, because it will teach you to be organised, structured and clear.

What to do with the 'difficult' patient

Some patients may, because of their mental disorder, be difficult to interview. If this is the case:

- Take the history as well as you can.
- Concentrate on completing as detailed a mental state examination as possible.

- Try to control your nerves. The examiners will have been told by the exam co-ordinator of your difficulties. Tell the examiners what happened (once).
- What they want is your considered professional opinion based on the information (however limited) available to you. Try to adjust your mindset so that this is what you offer them.
- Tell the examiners what you saw and heard, your current clinical opinion, what diagnoses could explain this presentation, your need for further information (state what you wish to learn, how you would seek this and your purpose in needing to know, etc.). You can still pass.

The vital quarter hour

Try to complete the basic history in approximately 45 minutes. In the remaining time check through your sheets while the patient is still in the room. There may (but not necessarily) be 5–10 minutes in addition before you go in to see the examiners after the patient is taken out of the room. This is an important time to gather your thoughts.

You do not have time to re-write or indeed read out the entire history for the examiners. Remember that the purpose of the history is to try to understand the person and their problems. You want to paint a picture for the examiners of the patient you have seen. Focus what you say in order to paint this picture effectively.

Structuring your presentation

Think in advance about the six areas you will be expected to cover:

1. Presentation of the history and mental state.
2. Differential diagnosis (with justifications).
3. Aetiology – the three Ps:
   - Predisposing factors.
   - Precipitating factors.
   - Perpetuating factors.

4. Investigations (social, psychological, physical).
5. Management (immediate and long-term; social, psychological, physical).
6. Prognosis (short-term, long-term).

Preparing to present the case

You have approximately 7–10 minutes to present the whole case. Of this, it is the opening few minutes that matter the most. It is during this time that you will present either a favourable or unfavourable impression. Examiners, being human, tend to label you as clearly passing or failing early on in the presentation. In our experience, it is quite difficult to switch between these labels once they are applied, therefore it is vital to have the 'right' label attached as soon as possible. How can you make this happen?

Prepare to pass

Prepare your opening few sentences. If the patient has been a difficult or poor historian say so now and possibly again later, but only once more. Do not overstate this. Next, **write out** the first two or three sentences of your presentation.

1. **A summary demographic statement**. Write this out in advance as one sentence only (see example below).
2. **The key problems** in the case. Write these out in advance as one or two sentences only (see example below).
   - What are the key problems?
   - You need to **focus** the history on these.
3. **Be ready to present the salient features of the whole history and mental state examination**.

Presenting the case

- State the **headings** whilst presenting the case in order to give clear signposts of where you are in the presentation ('Key features from the personal history include: . . .' etc.).

- Make sure that the flow of the history is **logical**, and present the history in a form that most examiners will recognise (see the discussion on taking the history above).
- Make sure that you communicate to the examiners that any important screening questions have been asked, even if there is no positive reply. For example 'On direct questioning there was no evidence of any of the first rank symptoms of schizophrenia', or 'There was evidence of early morning wakening, but no other biological symptoms of depression'.

Act of presentation

Remember:
- Keep calm.
- Modify the following suggested model to fit your cases. If you already have an effective structure of presentation that you are happy with, then don't change it too much unless you want to.
- Definitely do not change your regular style of presentation **on the day of the exam**. Get used to one style of presentation, and stick to it.
- Make your presentation interesting; it helps to vary your voice tone as you present, and to make good eye contact with both examiners.

The following summarises the structure of a typical presentation:

1. **A demographic summary sentence**.
   'The gentleman I saw is Mr S. J., who is a 33-year-old married man who lives alone in his own house.'

2. **One or two sentences summarising the key problem areas**.
   This is the main focus of the history. **Write this out in advance.**
   'He has had problems which began after the ending of his marriage four months ago. Since then he has been feeling **depressed**, **anxious** and **suicidal**. This led him to take an **overdose** that precipitated the admission to hospital. There are a number of associated difficulties including a lack of **social support** and isolation which have aggravated his situation.'

3. **Key parts of the rest of the history and mental state examination**.
   'He presented two weeks ago with . . ..'

   . . . then on to describe the main complaint (e.g. the depressive cluster of symptoms) and each of the other problem areas one by one.

- Read these from your history sheets.
- They should not need to be re-written.
- Go through the rest of the history reading out the relevant items. Draw attention to positive findings, and important negatives (e.g. first rank symptoms example as before).
- Use set phrases to save time: *'Mr S. J. describes a normal birth, development, childhood and schooling history. He left school at 16 and . . ..'.* This informs the examiners that you have asked about these areas, but without spending valuable time stating this in full.

Presentation of the history should paint a picture of the person, their problems and the aetiological factors. Mention the relevant **p**redisposing, **p**recipitating or **p**erpetuating factors as you go through the history. After presenting the salient points of the history and the mental state examination, you will move on to present the differential diagnosis.

The differential diagnosis

Consider both psychiatric and physical differential diagnoses.

- There may be no single right answer.
- 'There are a number of possibilities which include . . ..'.
  e.g. '. . . a range of psychiatric and physical disorders can cause a similar presentation. In this particular case I would consider X, Y and Z based on the following reasons . . ..'
- If it is obvious, however, state what you feel the diagnosis is.
- Show that you know that patients can change, and that your opinions are not fixed, but based upon the evidence that you find now at interview.

If it is very complicated, don't panic. Instead you can use a statement like: 'This is a very complicated case. After only an hour with the patient and without the chance to review the old notes or talk to an informant, I have a range of differential diagnoses, but at the present time I would not be able to put them into any definite order. However my differential diagnosis at present is . . .'.

- If someone appears guarded, always consider including paranoid psychosis in the differential diagnosis.

State the diagnosis you favour at the present time. Using information from the history make the case **for** and **against** each of the differential diagnoses in turn.

Standardised differential diagnoses

You will be required to use the ICD 10 classification in the exams. You should therefore familiarise yourself with this classification. It can be very helpful to have pre-prepared a list of 'standardised' differential diagnoses for the common presenting problems that you come across. These are not lists merely to regurgitate, but instead help you to remember the range of diagnostic possibilities (both psychiatric and physical) for you to consider. Having these to fall back on can be a great help if anxiety levels are high and you are finding it difficult to think effectively during the exam. Do remember to only state these if you **really are considering them** for this particular case.

Only state actual possibilities. Don't just say 'or an organic cause of the disorder'. You must be specific about what you have in mind, and give evidence to support it, e.g. 'Hypothyroidism, in view of the history of loss of energy and marked weight gain'.

Again, only state these if you **really are** considering them in the differential for this particular case. Be prepared to justify your reasons for and against each of your differential diagnoses.

Differential diagnosis of depression using ICD 10

1. **Bipolar affective disorder**
   - Specify type of current episode.
2. **Depressive episode**
   - Mild or moderate depressive episode +/– somatic symptoms.
   - Severe depressive episode +/– psychotic symptoms.
3. **Recurrent depressive disorder**
4. **Persistent mood disorders**
   - Dysthymia.
   - Cyclothymia.
5. **Adjustment disorder**
6. **Mixed affective episode**
7. **Personality disorder**
8. **Organic cause**
   - Hypothyroidism.
   - Alcohol dependence.
   - Other.

Differential diagnosis of paranoid ideas using ICD 10

1. Schizophrenia.
2. Schizotypal disorder.
3. Schizoaffective disorder.
4. Persistent delusional disorder.
5. Acute and transient psychotic disorders.
6. Personality disorder (schizoid or paranoid).
7. Mania with psychotic symptoms.
8. Bipolar affective disorder: manic or depressed +/– psychotic symptoms.
9. Severe depressive episode with psychotic features.
10. Recurrent depressive disorder: current episode severe with psychotic symptoms.
11. Organic cause:
    - Drug-induced/alcohol.
    - Temporal lobe epilepsy.
    - Other (systemic lupus erythematosus, third ventricular tumour, etc.).

Investigations

Social

Do not neglect this area. It is a very important part of good psychiatric practice.

- 'I would obtain the old notes and read them'.
- 'I would speak to a relative, with the patient's consent'.
- 'I would speak to the ward staff and ask do they eat, sleep, mix and laugh, etc.'.
- 'I would consider other sources of information: GP, Consultant, etc.'.
- Self-monitor: drinking or eating diary.
- Specialised reports can be requested if appropriate (e.g. social report, home visit, etc.).

Say **why** you would pursue each of these courses of action.

Psychological

Tests such as psychometric testing, mood rating scales, mood diaries, etc., may be indicated. Know how these are structured and how to use them. Make sure you know one ot two mood rating scales addressing anxiety, depression and social function.

Physical

Think out in advance which investigations are **appropriate** for each illness. 'These could include . . .' (see box on page 118).

Use your common sense – say what you do in **practice**.

Management

You need to show that you are competent, safe and sensible. It is important to say basic principles first even if they seem obvious:

- 'I would admit for a period of assessment' (if appropriate).
- 'I would want to treat each of their problems in turn . . .' etc.

- Bloods. State which and **why**. These could include full blood count (FBC), plasma viscosity (PV), renal, liver, calcium, sugar, vitamin B$_{12}$, folic acid, VDRL (venereal disease research laboratory) test and thyroid function tests (TFTs). Lithium levels may be appropriate. Know why these are performed, and the relevance if they reveal an abnormality.
- Urine drug analysis if appropriate.
- EEG if appropriate.
- Computerised tomography (CT) or MRI if appropriate.
- Blood alcohol levels if appropriate, etc.

Structured management plans

It is important to organise this part of the presentation in two ways:

1. Immediate and long-term management.
2. Physical, psychological and social aspects.

As part of your exam preparation you should **write out typical structured management plans for the core psychiatric conditions**. Include affective disorders, schizophrenia, neuroses, substance misuse, eating disorders, etc. Although you will have to present a management plan tailored to the individual case that you see on the day, this will be easier if you have previously prepared typical examples in this way.

Prognosis

State your experience, not just papers. Consider:

1. The **classical prognosis** of this condition: make sure that you have learned the typical prognosis for common disorders (schizophrenia, depression, mania, panic, alcoholism, etc.).
2. **Specific features** of this patient which affect it in this case:
   - Previous history.
   - Response to medication.
   - Concordance/compliance/adherence with treatment.
   - Social supports.

- Characteristics and personality strengths of the patient.
- Skills acquired.
- Degree of intelligence and willingness to work collaboratively with you on their problems.

Key points

The exam involves:

- Meeting a patient for the first time and winning his/her confidence.
- Obtaining a fully structured and relevant history.
- The physical examination should be brief and concentrate especially on areas that will aid in establishing a diagnosis.
- Planning your investigations and management according to your differential diagnosis.
- Making sure that you come over as safe, sensible and professional.

REFERENCES

1. Gelder M, Lopez-Ibor JH, Andraesen NC (2003) *New Oxford Textbook of Psychiatry*. Oxford University Press: Oxford.
2. Williams CJ (2001) *Overcoming Depression: A Five Area Approach*. Hodder Arnold Publishers: London.

Presenting the individual patient assessment (IPA) to the examiners (Part II)

Peter Trigwell and Christopher Williams

The clinical assessment with the examiners lasts for 30 minutes. There will usually be two College examiners there when you present your long clinical case (also known as the individual patient assessment or IPA). Do not be worried if a third (the external examiner) is sitting in the background. He or she is present merely to record whether the performance of the examiners appears reliable and valid. He or she will make no contribution at all to your final mark, which is decided by the two main examiners alone.

Presentation techniques

- Passing the long case clinical exam (IPA) involves presenting yourself well.
- Go in and act confidently.
- Do not say your name. State your **examination number** when asked (have it written down).
- Be polite and professional. Do not come over as too eager to please.
- Make eye contact with both examiners as you start presenting, **and** subsequently.
- If the examiners enquire about something that you have forgotten to ask the patient about, say that you would have normally enquired about this and why it would be important **in this case**.
- Don't shuffle the papers too much.

It is important to be adaptive and flexible. Carefully consider any suggestions the examiners make to you about diagnosis, etc. Do not reject any suggestions they make out of hand, but show that you can consider the evidence for and against a particular diagnostic possibility. The patient's presentation may have changed since the history was summarised for the examiners, or the patient may now be partially treated or have relapsed. Also, remember the clinical effects of medication or ECT on the mental state.

Difficult questions in the long case

Certain questions are often dreaded by candidates. This is unnecessary as they can be tackled in a straightforward and systematic way.

1. 'Present a psychodynamic formulation'

Sometimes an examiner will ask you to present a psychodynamic formulation of your case. Do not be thrown by this. You already have all the information that you require to answer this in your case history. Consider the person's:

a) **Mother and father** – their relationship with each parent; any evidence of excessive dependency or hostility, etc; any separation/individuation issues.

b) **Personal history** – important issues/factors that stand out as being psychodynamically relevant, e.g. perceived abandonment or rejection; repeating patterns in relationships, etc.

c) **Defence mechanisms** – have any obvious defence mechanisms (e.g. projection, denial, etc.) been used in the past? Look for continuity of these defence mechanisms over time.

d) **Features at interview** – any obvious defence mechanisms present during the interview; these may include avoiding painful issues, or crying when particular issues are touched upon; consider both conscious coping mechanisms and unconscious ego defence mechanisms; consider the patient's reaction to you (transference), and also your reactions to the patient (counter-transference).

e) **Keep your formulation simple** – address it to the specific patient; say why these features are important, e.g. in considering treatment.

2. 'Describe this person's personality'

Again, this question is not as difficult as it may seem. Apart from describing the patient's main personality traits you must comment upon three areas:

a) In your experience, is their personality normal or abnormal?
b) If it is abnormal, do they cause themselves or others to suffer? (i.e. do they have a personality disorder?)
c) If they do have a personality disorder, which one is it in ICD 10?

To do this well, you need to know the ICD 10 diagnostic criteria. If the patient's characteristics do not fully satisfy any of the criteria (as is often the case) say so:

'They do not exactly fulfil the criteria for any specific personality disorder. However they show aspects of certain ICD 10 personality disorders including. . . '.

3. 'Carry out a CBT formulation'

For example, using the five areas assessment CBT approach[1]:

a) **Situation, relationship or practical problems faced** – what situations cause symptoms? (e.g. going into a shop alone leads to panic); consider the social situation, their supports and practical problems faced such as debt, unemployment and housing problems.
b) **Altered thinking** – how do they interpret what happens? (e.g. what are their fears during the panic attack?); identify any extreme and unhelpful thoughts; identify possible core beliefs or unhelpful rules, e.g. 'I'm worthless/bad/unlovable . . .', 'Others let you down', etc.; identify any possible unhelpful thinking styles[1] (bias against themselves, jumping to conclusions, catastrophic thinking, mind-reading, etc.).
c) **Altered feelings** – anxiety; depression; anger; shame; guilt, etc.
d) **Altered physical/physiological changes** – biological symptoms in depression; arousal symptoms in anxiety/panic.
e) **Altered activity/behaviour/impact** – e.g. reducing or stopping doing things in depression and withdrawal; reduced pleasure and sense of achievement as a result; avoidance and safety behav-

iours in anxiety and unhelpful behaviours such as drinking as a
way of blocking how they feel.

The five areas assessment

The five areas approach[1] is an NHS-sponsored development of CBT
to 'translate' CBT into a user-friendly model for use with patients. It
is supported by two books addressing depression and anxiety (generalised anxiety, panic/phobias, obsessive-compulsive disorder and
health problems) that are aimed at teaching practitioners and
patients core CBT skills and interventions that can be used in everyday clinical practice.

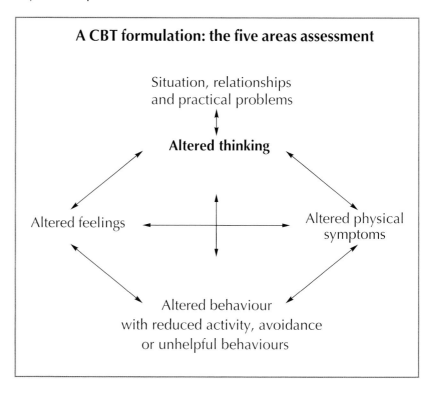

A CBT formulation: the five areas assessment

Situation, relationships
and practical problems

Altered thinking

Altered feelings

Altered physical
symptoms

Altered behaviour
with reduced activity, avoidance
or unhelpful behaviours

Interviewing in front of the examiners

During the IPA in Part II of the exam, you will be required to interview the patient in front of the examiners for approximately 5–10 minutes. The purpose of this is to allow the examiners to gauge:

- Your professionalism.
- Your manner with the patient (tact and empathy).
- Your clinical skills as a psychiatrist (listening skills, objectivity, interviewing skills).
- Your ability to elicit and demonstrate psychopathology (goal-directed approach, phrasing of questions, etc.).

Many candidates find this a most stressful experience. It is rarely practised beforehand and, as a result, is a potential 'weak spot'. It is essential to practise this part of the exam under examination conditions. It may be possible to do this within the setting of ward rounds but it is better to do it as a separate exercise. You need to discover your potential weaknesses, and work to improve them. Ask yourself:

- 'Do I come over as a professional doctor with good clinical skills?'
- 'Do I show myself to be a warm, genuine listener, and at the same time can I take charge and direct the clinical interview?'
- 'Can I work efficiently to gather specific information in a clear way?'
- 'Which clinical symptoms do I find the most difficult to phrase questions about?'

The examiners want to know if you can control the interview, ask clinical questions competently and structure your time to complete the task in the time allocated, whilst being professional and polite to the patient. You must also come over as being genuine. If you have problems with being warm and empathic do not over-compensate. This is likely to appear false. You will be far better off in this circumstance if you adopt a professional manner that is polite but not brusque.

Typical questions the examiners may ask you with the patient present

There are certain questions which can be answered well in 5–10 minutes, and so are often asked:

1. **Fact gathering**
   - 'Take a full alcohol history'.
   - 'Assess the suicide risk'.

2. **Eliciting symptoms**
   - 'Can you ask about their ideas concerning cleanliness and try to show whether this reflects an obsessional illness or not?'
   - 'You mentioned that at times they feel threatened by those around them. Can you please ask a little more to try and decide whether these ideas are delusional?'

3. **Confirm or refute a diagnosis**
   - 'You mentioned earlier that it is possible the presentation may be caused by schizophrenia. Can you ask the patient more to try and examine this diagnosis in greater detail?'

4. **Specific task**
   - 'Test the cognitive state of the patient' (or specified parts of this). The Mini Mental State Examination[3] is a useful short test to use in these circumstances.
   - 'Can you test the orientation and short- (or) long-term memory of the patient please?'

Techniques

- Remember you have done this many times before.
- **Write down the questions the examiners wish you to cover.** If you are uncertain, ask for clarification.
- Set up the chairs that you and the patient will sit in so that they are at an angle to each other of about 90 degrees and a comfortable distance apart, reflecting your knowledge of good interview technique.

- Bring in the patient and introduce him or her to the examiners.
- Show the patient to their chair.
- Set the scene to the patient in front of the examiners. Show that you are aware that this is stressful for the patient as well. Try to help the patient relax and put them at ease. Say something like: '**Thank you** for coming in. It's **important** for me to be able to talk to you in front of the examiners for the purposes of this exam. Try to **relax** if you can, because it's me who is under the spotlight today, rather than you. I want to start by asking you **some questions which we've covered already**, but if you'll just bear with me it will only take **about 5 or 10 minutes** . . . Well, I'd like to start by asking you . . .'.
- Some examiners are irritated if you are too familiar with the patient. You should always refer to them as Mr, Miss, Ms or Mrs, etc., and not address them by their first name unless they ask you to do so.
- Make sure that you cover all the questions that you were asked to.
- **Start from first principles**. Do not refer to things the patient has already told you during your first meeting with them. This can cause you to ask them very leading questions, and shows poor technique, e.g. 'I would like to ask you one or two further questions about the problems with checking that you mentioned earlier'.
- Make it obvious to the examiners which questions you are answering. If you feel that you are 'stuck' on an area, you can always move on and justify your decision later to the examiners. 'I have a number of things that the examiners want me to cover in only a few minutes, so we'll have to move on from this area'.
- **Try to ask open questions first, followed by more closed questions, as indicated by the patient's answers.**
- If the examiners have asked you to check whether a particular symptom is present do this quickly and efficiently. For example, if you are asked to elicit a belief and see if it is delusion (i.e. a fixed, false and unshakeable belief), then you must try and demonstrate that this is the case, with the belief being maintained in the face of logical argument and evidence to the contrary, or that the belief is based on delusional evidence.

- **Decide on the ordering and prioritising of the questions**. For example, if you are asked to assess the long- and the short-term memory of the person, you should reverse the order of the questions so that you can give information to test short-term memory (e.g. 'I am going to tell you a short address . . .') at the **start** of the interview rather than at the end. This avoids an uncomfortable two minute wait at the end of the interview before you can test their recall of the address. As long as you ensure that you cover all the required areas, you can carry out the tasks in whatever order you think is best.
- Don't worry if the patient does not give the answer that you expect. Ask again in a different way. If at the end of a reasonable selection of questions things still seem unclear, move on. You can always be honest and tell the examiners if they ask you whether you felt you carried out an adequate assessment. If you feel you have not been able to confirm or refute the symptom, then you could for example say: 'I didn't feel that based on the replies that the patient gave there was evidence of thought disorder. I would want to spend more time with him/her to check this further'.
- At the end of the interview, thank the patient again and show them out of the room.

After the patient has left, the examiners may ask you what you noticed, and whether you were happy that you elicited the information adequately. Be objective in your reply. They may also ask whether any new information has been unearthed which may influence your differential diagnosis or management. If this is the case say so, again showing that you are able to take account of and integrate new information.

The present state examination

One of the worries that candidates often have is 'How should I ask appropriate questions?' Make sure you know how to ask about the presence of:

1. Psychotic symptoms:

- Hallucinations
- Delusions

2. 'Neurotic' symptoms:
  - Depersonalisation/derealisation
  - Worry
  - Anxiety
  - Panic attacks
  - Obsessions/compulsions
  - Hypochondriasis

Most people find that it is the 'psychotic' questions that are the hardest to phrase, as well as those asking about depersonalisation. Practise these in your everyday history-taking. If you are uncertain how to phrase the questions, look at questions used in the 'Present State Examination' (Wing et al[4]). These start with 'open' questions, have been widely used in clinical research settings, and have been found to be reliable. Many previous candidates have found these standardised questions very helpful.

Typical PSE questions include:

1. Delusional mood:
   - 'Have you ever had the feeling that something odd is going on that you can't explain?'
   - 'What is it like?'

2. Depersonalisation:
   - 'Have you felt recently as if the world is unreal, or only an imitation of reality, like a stage set?'
   - 'Have you felt that you yourself are not a real person, not really part of the living world, like an actor playing a part?'

3. Delusions of reference and persecution:
   - 'Have you felt that people are unduly interested in you, or that things are arranged so as to have a special meaning?'
   - 'Does anyone seem to be trying to harm you (trying to poison or kill you)?'

Key points

- **Write down** the areas you are asked to cover by the examiners.
- Be confident and take charge (arrange the chairs, etc.).
- Show the patient in and introduce him/her to the examiners.
- Show the patient to their seat and set the scene for him/her.
- If possible use PSE questions. Obtain a list of these before the exam and learn the most 'difficult' ones (e.g. depersonalisation).
- Elicit what was asked for. **Open** questioning is best, leading on to closed questioning.
- Impose your own structure and prioritise your asking of the questions as you think is best.
- Be polite and courteous at all times.
- Thank the patient again and show him/her out.

REFERENCES

1. Williams CJ (2001) *Overcoming Depression: A Five Areas approach.* Arnold Publishers: London.

2. Williams CJ (2003) *Overcoming Anxiety: A Five Areas approach.* Arnold Publishers: London.

3. Folstein MF, Folstein SE, McHugh PR (1975) Mini-mental state. A practical method for grading the cognitive state of patients for the clinician. *Journal of Psychiatric Research* 12 (3): 189–198.

4. Wing JK, Cooper JE, Sartorius N (1974) *Measurement and Classification of Psychiatric Symptoms.* Cambridge University Press: Cambridge.

Patient management problems (PMPs – the clinical vignettes)

Christopher Williams

Patient management problems (PMPs, also called clinical vignettes) occur in the Part II examination only. They are set by a second pair of examiners, and take place at the same centre and on the same day as the long case individual patient assessment. The exam lasts 30 minutes and consists of three PMP questions. For each vignette candidates will be assessed on an 11 point scale ranging from 10 (excellent) to 0 (very poor). A grade of 5 or more is required for a Pass in the PMP.

It is important to practise this part of the exam. Many candidates find them surprisingly difficult, simply because they have not become familiar with the technique. In reality, all you have to say is essentially what you would do in best practice and show that you can answer questions sensibly and appropriately. You have solved similar problems whilst 'on call' for the last few years and the key to success in this part of the exam is harnessing this experience as well as your wider academic knowledge.

You will be expected to answer with a level of knowledge that could reasonably be expected of someone after 2.5 years of training in psychiatry. Do not be put off if a question is put to you by an examiner who you fear may be a specialist in the area of the question they ask. For example, if you have never done child psychiatry do not be perturbed by questions such as 'How would you treat urinary incontinence in a child by using the Star chart method?'. All that will be expected is for you to have a reasonable overall level of knowledge, and to understand the general principles involved.

What are examiners looking for?

Vignettes are written in advance by a range of examiners. They are not made up on the day by the individual examiners. Each vignette addresses a real-life clinical problem and should last no more than 10 minutes. All the necessary clinical information you require to answer the question should be given in the vignette. Usually examiners will present a brief outline of a case in a few sentences, and will then ask you up to three questions that will require you to explore different aspects of the problem. The examiners want to assess your understanding of clinical issues, including the evidence base and especially whether you can think broadly and systematically in your answers. Be sure to show a competent and systematic problem solving approach to management.

> ## Key point
> You will need to show more than simple factual knowledge to gain a pass mark. You will also need to show that you have addressed a range of the key issues. PMP vignettes are each designed to highlight five areas of knowledge, at least three of which must be mentioned in order to pass. Examiners have a pre-written 'template' answer identifying a range of the key issues you might be expected to provide – however they can mark your answer flexibly so as to add marks if you identify additional relevant areas.

PMP techniques

It is therefore essential to be **systematic** and **organised** in your approach to answering PMPs. As the examiners ask you the question, try to identify the key issues/main problem areas. You may wish to jot these down on a piece of paper and make sure you address each of these during your answer. It is important, however, not to restrict your answers to only one area or aspect of the problem, thus going down a 'blind alley' and running out of things to say. Keep your answers broad. You need to have a clear:

- Opening.
- Middle: impose a structure/keep it broad.
- Ending: come to a clear end.

Opening

Try to avoid a lengthy pause. Your answer should have a clear opening. The following **three approaches** may help you start and structure your answer.

1. Key issues

What are the main issues raised by the question?

- Safety/risk issues.
- Issues of diagnosis.
- Management.
- Any Mental Health Act/Common Law issues?

'This question involves a number of different issues. These include the importance of being sure of the original diagnosis, the need for a full assessment, and also the difficulties of treating those with treatment resistant depression . . ..'

This has the advantage of showing the examiners that you can pick out the **key points/problem areas** quickly and have a firm grasp of the essentials of care. When you use this approach, make sure that you start off by describing the most relevant or important problem area first in order to avoid interruptions by impatient examiners.

2. Further information needed

Do you need any more information? Where from?

- To make the diagnosis.
- To decide on treatment.
- To assess the impact on the patient: what has he/she stopped doing because of the problem?
- To assess the impact on other people (e.g. carers, etc.).

'In this case I would wish to gather **further information** in order to clarify the diagnosis. I would talk to x,y,z in order to find out . . ..'

3. 'Talk yourself into the situation'
Imagine you have been asked to deal with this clinical problem whilst on call. What would you do in practice?

'If I was asked to go and see this case in casualty, I would begin thinking about how to manage the case on the way there. I would first go to the Medical Records Office, look up and obtain their old notes and quickly read them in order to find out more information. I would also phone the ward where they had been an inpatient and see if any of the nursing staff knew them . . ..'

Some people find this approach is most effective if you use visual imagery whilst talking about how you would deal with the situation. **This approach is often particularly helpful if you are feeling quite anxious.**

Do not begin to answer each question in exactly the same way. This may annoy and frustrate the examiners.

The middle/main component

Keep your thinking **broad**. Consider using different perspectives in your answer to aid this.

- Remember to consider **psychological** and **social** aspects of the diagnosis and treatment as well as **physical** ones (e.g. effects on the patient, their family and work).
- What are the benefits and risks of treatment?
- Consider immediate and long-term treatment.
- Consider additional assessments/reviews during interventions – which would include both the patient and also family, carers and friends who know the person and are providing important support (with the patient's consent).

Remember that as you answer you are providing cues that will stimulate further questions from your examiners. Use this wisely. Try to avoid digging yourself into a hole.

Ending and possible problems

- Come to a clear end and look up, waiting for the next question/clarification.

Potential difficulties in answering PMPs

If you do not know part of an answer, say where you would go for appropriate and sensible advice. For example, if you do not know what drugs you can safely prescribe in pregnancy it is reasonable to say, 'I would contact Pharmacy and Drug Information and ask for further information'.

If the examiners appear to disagree with you strongly, be prepared to consider other possibilities. Feel able to discuss other diagnostic or treatment options. **Never get into an argument**, but if you think that you are correct, you should review with the examiners the reasons for and against each of the possibilities, and the reasons why you wish for the time being to stick to your first decision. Always show that if more information became available, or the person changed, you would be willing to reconsider.

The principles of effective answering of PMPs are illustrated by the following examples. Variants of these questions are commonly asked in the exam. Lists of many previously asked PMPs are summarised on widely used examination resource websites:

Web-based resources

www.superego-cafe.com
www.trickcyclists.co.uk
www.mrcpsych.com
www.psychejam.com
www.mrcpsych-help.com
www.fiveareas.com (a site designed to support this book)

Example: treatment resistant depression

'A 65-year-old man has been weepy and depressed for 3 months. He has lost significant weight and there is marked anhedonia. He has been treated with fluoxetine for the last 8 weeks and continues to be very low in mood. He has begun to express ideas of hopelessness and is feeling suicidal.'

The examiners may ask questions such as the following. These are usually given consecutively to test the depth of your knowledge as you answer.

- How would you manage this patient?
- Would you make any change of medication? If so, what would you do and why?
- You make all these changes and he continues to be unwell. How would you manage him now?

Spend about 5 minutes answering this question by jotting down your answers on a piece of paper. Try to be **organised** as you answer. What are the **main points** you need to cover?

- What are the main issues in this case?
- What further information might you need?

Possible components of the answer
Opening

1. Main issues, e.g.:
   - How to manage treatment resistant depression.
   - Treatment issues in older patients.
   - The need to clarify the diagnosis.

2. Further information needed, e.g.:
   - Is it a depressive disorder?
   - Is there a co-morbidity (physical or psychiatric)?
   - Concordance/compliance issues, etc.

3. Talk yourself into the situation: 'If I was seeing this patient for the first time in clinic . . .'.

Middle/main component of your answer

Expand on the areas mentioned in Opening 1 (main issues involved) or 2 (information needed).

Is the diagnosis correct?

In a 65-year-old man with weight loss, perhaps there is a hidden physical disorder (such as cancer). Has this been excluded?

'I would want to confirm that the diagnosis **actually is depression**. I would do both a full psychiatric history and also a detailed mental state examination. I would examine the person physically and send off appropriate screening bloods for physical disease. In particular, I would send off a full blood count to check for anaemia, and thyroid function tests to exclude thyroid disorder. If any other physical tests are warranted, I would request these (e.g. a chest X-ray in a smoker).'

Check current and past management

*   Ask other obvious questions: 'Is he actually taking the fluoxetine?'
*   'Is he taking an appropriate dose for an adequate time?'

'I would want to know if he was taking the tablets at an adequate dose. Within BNF guidelines, I would increase the dose as far as could be tolerated by the patient . . ..'

Gather more information to make sure

State the information you require, how you would obtain it, and why you want to know:

'I would also obtain the old notes and read them. It would be helpful to talk to an informant, with the patient's permission. I would like to get a clear description from nursing staff, etc., of how the patient is during the day to see if his behaviour is consistent with a diagnosis of depression.'

One important focus of this question is 'How do you treat resistant depression?'. This is a classic and often repeated PMP. Make sure you have planned answers to such common management difficulties.

Do not neglect to mention **maintaining factors**. It is easy in a question such as this to only mention physical approaches to treatment. Abnormal personality, alcohol or substance misuse, and ongoing social and relationship problems are potential maintaining factors for depression as can be concurrent physical illness or even treatments such as anti-hypertensive medication or the use of steroids. These would need to be addressed. The reactions of family members may also be relevant.

Ending

• Make it clear when you have finished your response.

The examiners may then either go on to another PMP, or add a further stem to the current question which will introduce a fresh angle to the problem. It is important to remember that there are a number of ways of answering any PMP. What matters most is that you are seen to be safe and sensible.

Practising PMPs with a local consultant or SpR can be helpful in preparing for the PMP exam. If you are confused by the question, be honest and say so. It is far better to clarify the question than to attempt it without understanding what is being asked.

Key points
Opening
• Have a clear opening using one of the three techniques outlined above ('main issues', 'further information needed', or 'talk yourself into the situation') and gain thinking time by concentrating on the key issues of the case.
• Don't use the same opening approach for each question.
• Be aware of the range of possible questions.

Middle

- Organise your answer clearly.
- Demonstrate that you are sensible and safe.
- Say what you would do in practice.
- Be divergent in your thinking and avoid going down a blind alley. Address each of the main problem areas.
- Use techniques to keep your answer **broad** and **organised** (e.g. short- and long-term management; treatment benefits and risks; physical, psychological and social management options).
- Show that you are **flexible** and will consider the evidence for and against a range of diagnostic or treatment options if this is appropriate.
- Where appropriate, say that you would seek advice or information from others with more experience in that area.

Ending

- Come to a clear end.

Remember: Do not be dogmatic and where appropriate say that you would seek advice or information from others with more experience in that area.

If at first you don't succeed . . .

Kevin Appleton

Failing the exam

Not everyone passes the MRCPsych. Many people will have sat the exam one or more times previously. Failure will be experienced by a large number of candidates at some time whilst trying to pass both parts of the MRCPsych exam. I was such a person. This short section is dedicated to those people who may have a similar experience to me at some time. There are those who work long and hard, apparently covering all the topics thoroughly, but who still fail. This is a most disheartening experience and can cause a myriad of feelings including upset, and anger.

It is difficult to alleviate the sense of disappointment and exhaustion that follows the receipt of your application forms for the next attempt and condolences from the chief examiner. At this stage try to send off the form to **request feedback on your performance** as soon as possible. It is easy to be so fed up that you feel you never want to do the exam again. You may adopt an attitude somewhat akin to 'learned helplessness'. Failure will trigger off many thoughts that will convince you that Beck's Negative Cognitive Triad is an accurate model of depression. You are likely to feel pessimistic about yourself, the world and the future. You may begin to make negative predictions, and have the most catastrophic thoughts about the exam or your career. As with all such thoughts, they are both unhelpful and inaccurate.

Sending off for feedback can actually help challenge these beliefs.

It can show you that **you are not bad at every part of the exam**. Realising this can be quite encouraging. You will have done better on some parts of the exam than others. This is useful information, because it shows you which areas of your performance you need to change.

Next is the difficult task of giving the bad news to others. Everyone wants to know if you passed but no one wants to ask you. Your colleagues may study you intensely from a distance to pick up clues (drooping shoulders, dishevelled appearance) before deciding whether to sit with you at lunch. Some people do genuinely wish to hear all about it and may allow you to off-load your sorrows. For others, try using a brief but positive sound bite.

At some stage you do need to accept the fact that failing an exam is a kind of bereavement. You need to give yourself time to recover before starting again. Try to be good to yourself, get plenty of sleep, and go out and do some of your favourite things. Do something different which is fun (and non-psychiatric). A short holiday away, or booking on to a course you have always wanted to do can be useful. There may also be practical matters that have been neglected during the intense revision and that need to be caught up with. Dealing with these will take your mind off the exam and put things in perspective. Family and friends may have had less of your time and attention recently, so take the opportunity to remedy this. They need to have you back for a while and you need their support and encouragement. Try to move your focus away from just the exam; in the long term failing the exam will not seem so important. No one in their right mind would choose to fail but if it happens it isn't the end of the world.

Looking to the future

You will have to try and work out exactly what did go wrong in your performance, and start to plan a strategy for another attempt. At a fairly early stage you should decide whether you are going to resit at the next opportunity or wait 6 months or more. This decision will have to be based on a number of factors. These may include practical matters such as house moves or any other foreseeable events that might make it just too difficult to give enough time to your revision. If possible, applying to resit soon is probably the best thing to do for two reasons. First, it helps you maintain momentum. Even if you take 6 or 8 weeks off from learning after the last exam, your previous revision will be relatively fresh in your memory. You can use this as a firm foundation to build on. Secondly, there is only a short window of opportunity where you are allowed to apply for the exam. If you miss it, you will not be able to apply for the next sitting. If you are in doubt it is often best to apply and secure a place. For many people motivation to work comes back slowly with time, and this can be accelerated by having the focus (and financial commitment) of a booked exam. If you change your mind later, you can always choose to withdraw prior to the exam without this being counted as an attempt. There will be a financial penalty for doing this, however, as outlined in the College application forms.

The initial feedback from the College will tell you which part of the exam you have failed. The later feedback (which you have to request), may not arrive until a few weeks before the next exam. Do not wait until you receive this to go to see your clinical tutor, consultant, or other helpful persons who can help you at your next attempt. If you don't already belong to a study group this may also be the time to get together with three or four like-minded people who intend to take the exam at the next sitting. These groups can be a great source of support, encouragement, shared learning and knowledge.

After failing Part II, I felt that although I possessed a lot of theoretical and practical knowledge about psychiatry, I had not used or communicated this well in the exam itself. My second attempt involved a much greater emphasis on technique, after attending the Leeds MRCPsych Examination Technique course. Much useful work was also done in study group gatherings. This helped to focus my learning on exam-relevant information, and I would recommend it.

Index

Notes

Page numbers followed by 'f' indicate figures.

In order to save space in the index the following abbreviations have been used:

CRP – critical review paper

EMI – extended matched items

IPA – individual patient assessment

ISQs – individual statement questions

OSCE – objective structured clinical examination

PMP – patient management problems

A

absolute risk reduction (ARR) 73

actors, in OSCE 42

adjustment disorder 116

affective disorders 116

  IPA 104

  OSCE 32–33

agoraphobia 30, 104

alcohol abuse/dependence

  IPA 104, 126

    mock clinical exams 102

  OSCE 30

analytical statistics 51, 60

ANOVA (analysis of variance) 60, 61

antidepressant therapy (explanation to patient) 30, 36–38

antipsychotic medication 94

anxiety (candidate, exam-related) 4, 22

anxiety disorders

  IPA 104, 129

    clustering symptoms 109–110

    mock clinical exams 102

  OSCE 30, 33

application deadlines 3

ARR (absolute risk reduction) 73

B

basic sciences MCQ paper 5, 11, 16, 17

bias 63, 64–65

  elimination 71, 76

bipolar affective disorder 116

blank questions 22

blinding 72

blood tests 118

BNF (*British National Formulary*) 10

brainstorming 91
British Journal of Psychiatry 84
British National Formulary
  (BNF) 10
bullet points 99

C
calculated guesswork 20
calculators 48
capacity assessment/manage-
  ment 30, 33
cardiopulmonary resuscitation,
  assessment 28, 35
case control studies 74–76
categorical data 50, 51
CBT (cognitive behavioural
  therapy) 34
CBT formulation 123–124
Central Office for Research
  Ethics Committees 72
CER (control event rate) 73
child and adolescent psychiatry
  17
Chi-squared test 51, 78
clinical examination skills
  IPA 105–107
  OSCE 35
clinical significance, definition
  63
clinical topics MCQ paper
  16, 17
clinical vignettes *see* patient
  management problems (PMPs)
clustering symptoms 109–110
cognitive assessment/manage-
  ment 30, 33

cognitive behavioural therapy
  (CBT) 34
  formulation 123–124
cognitive model of panic 14
cohort studies 74–76
*College Regulations for the
  MRCPsych Examinations* 1, 2
communication skills
  IPA 101
  OSCE 30, 42
concurrent validity 70
condensing information
  9–10, 19
confidence (in candidates) 20
confidence intervals 52, 64
confounding bias 65
confounding variables 65, 71
CONSORT guidelines 71
construct validity 70
content validity 69–70
continuing professional development 93, 97
control event rate (CER) 73
convergent validity 70
Core Psychiatry 10
correlation coefficients 61
Cox regression model 62
CPR assessment/technique
  28, 35
cranial nerve examination
  30, 35
criterion validity 70
Critical Appraisal for Psychiatry
  46
critical appraisal skills 4, 45, 47
critical review paper (CRP)
  4, 45–57

knowledge/skills required 47
research methods 48–49
revision topics 59–81
  case control and cohort
    studies 74–76
  RCTs 70–73
  screening and diagnosis
    66–70
  statistical terms 60–62,
    62–66
  statistical tests 50–52,
    60–62
  systematic reviews and
    meta-analysis 76–77
techniques 47–48
Critical Reviews in Psychiatry 46
cross validity 70
CRP see critical review paper
  (CRP)

D
data
  distribution 50–51, 61
  interpretation skills 30, 35,
    50–52
  types 50, 51, 60
deadlines, exam applications 3
degrees of freedom 51
delusions 39, 127, 129
depersonalisation 129
depression
  assessment/management
    OSCE 32
    symptom clustering
      108–109
  differential diagnosis 116
  ISQs 13

mock clinical exams 102
  treatment resistant 136–138
descriptive statistics 50–51, 60
Diabetes Prevention Research
  Group 95
diagnostic skills 103, 108–110
diagrams 99
differential diagnoses 114–116
'difficult' patients 110–111
discontinuation syndrome 37
distribution-free tests 51
divergent validity 70
double-spacing 99

E
eating disorders 102, 104
  assessment/management 33
  history taking 30
economic analysis 80
EER (experimental event rate) 73
effect size 73
emergency management 30, 35
EMIs *see* extended matched
  items (EMIs)
environmental factors, revision
  strategies 8
epidemiology, basic sciences
  MCQ paper 17
essays 83–100
  blindspots 100
  examiner's role 98
  layout 99
  preparation 84, 85
  referencing 99
  structuring 85–93, 99
    expansion techniques
      86–87

helicoptering 86, 86f, 89
tables/diagrams 99
topic identification 84–85
writing, web-based resources 87
writing process 93–97
ethics 72
ethology, basic sciences MCQ paper 17
Evidence-based Medicine 46
Evidence-based Mental Health 46
evidence-based practice 52
examination structure 1–3
see also specific elements
examination technique 6
CRP 47–48
EMIs 21–22
IPA 121–122
ISQs 21–22
MCQ paper *see* MCQ exams
PMPs 132–134
exam stress 4, 22
expansion techniques, essay structuring 86–87
experimental event rate (EER) 73
extended matched items (EMIs) 13
contents 16
definition 14
formulation/terminology 24
as revision aids 18
scoring 14–15
technique 21–22
'eyeball' funnel plot 79

F
face validity 56, 69
failure 141–143
'false' questions 20–21, 23
feedback 104, 141–142
finger agnosia 40
five areas assessment 123–124
fixed effects modelling 79
Forest Plots 77
Fundoscopy station, OSCE 28

G
Galbraith plot 79
Gaussian distribution 51, 61
general adult psychiatry 17
genetics 17
global learning style 7
group support 9
guesswork 20

H
hallucinations 39, 129
handwriting 98, 99
health anxiety 104
Health Professions Council (HPC) 90
helicoptering, essay structuring 86, 86f, 89
heterogeneity 79
history taking
IPA 103, 106–107, 111
OSCE 29, 30, 38–39
H_o (null hypothesis) 63
holistic learning style 7
How to Read a Paper 46

HPC (Health Professions Council) 90
human development 17
hyperventilation 110
hypochondriasis 104, 129

I

ICD 10 classification 10, 115–116, 123
illegible scripts 98, 99
inception cohort 74
inclusion bias 76, 79
incremental validity 70
individual patient assessment (IPA) 2, 4
  case preparation 101–119
    clinical assessment 105–107
    diagnosis 108–110, 114–116
    'difficult' patients 110–111
    history taking 103, 106–107, 111
    investigations 117
    management 117–118
    mock clinical exams 102–104
    physical examination 107
    predicting and practising cases 104–105
    prognosis 118–119
    structuring 111–112
  case presentation 112–114, 121–130
    CBT formulation approach 123–124
    difficult questions 122–124

    five areas assessment 124
    patient interviews 125–128
    present state examination 128–130
    'psychodynamic formulation' 122
    structure 111–112
    techniques 103, 121–122
individual statement questions (ISQs)
  contents 15, 16
    'true' and 'false' questions/ answers 20–21, 23
  definition 13
  formulation/terminology 23–24
  as revision aids 18
  scoring 14–15
  technique 21–22
information bias 65
information condensing 9–10, 19
information sources 10–11
  web-based *see* web-based resources
informed consent 72
insight assessment 34
intention to treat analysis 71
interval data 50, 60
interviewing patients 103, 125–128
Introduction to Psychotherapy 10
IPA *see* individual patient assessment (IPA)
ISQs *see* individual statement questions (ISQs)

J
journal articles 84
journal clubs 47

K
Kaplan Meier survival analysis 62
Kruskal–Wallis ANOVA 60

L
law (principles of), basic sciences MCQ paper 17
'lead-ins' 14
learning styles 4, 7–9
likelihood ratio 55, 67, 68f
lithium
    pharmacology 32, 118
    treatment 30
Liverpool University Neuroleptic Side Effect Rating Scale (LUNSERS) 96
location bias 76, 79
logistic regression 62
long case clinical examination *see* individual patient assessment (IPA)
LUNSERS (Liverpool University Neuroleptic Side Effect Rating Scale) 96

M
Mann-Whitney U test 51, 60
marking schemes 14–17, 31
MCQ exams 4, 13–26
    basic sciences paper 5, 11, 16, 17
    clinical topics paper 16, 17

EMIs *see* extended matched items (EMIs)
ISQs *see* individual statement questions (ISQs)
    marking scheme 14–17
    preparation 18–19
    structure 14–17
    technique 21–26
        terminology 24
        timing 21–22
    web-based resources 11
mean 50, 60
median 50, 60
medical classification 87–89
medical ethics 17
memory impairment 29, 30, 38–39
mental health (of candidates) 4, 22
mental state examination 29, 103, 114, 126
meta-analysis 76–80
Mind Maps™ 10
Mini Mental State Examination 126
mixed affective episode 116
mock clinical exams 102–104
mode 50, 60
mood disorders 116
mood rating scales 117
motivation (of candidates) 8–9
multiple choice questions (MCQs)
    as revision aids 18–19
    see also MCQ exams
multiple regression 62
multivariate analysis 60

N

negative predictive value (NPV)
55, 67
neuroleptic malignant syndrome 35
neurosciences 17
neurotic symptoms 129
NNT (number needed to treat)
73
nominal data 50, 60
nomogram 68, 68f
non-parametric tests 51
note-taking 9–10, 19
NPV (negative predictive value)
55
null hypothesis 63
number needed to treat (NNT)
73

O

objective structured clinical
examination (OSCE) 1, 27–43
antidepressant therapy explanation 30, 36–38
content 28–30
duration 29
marking scheme 31
memory impairment history
38–39
parietal lobe function 40–41
rationale 27
revision strategies 32–35
stations 28–30
strategy (on the day) 41–43
web-based resources 32
observer bias 64

obsessive-compulsive disorder
129
mock clinical exams 102, 104
odds ratio 75, 76, 79
old age psychiatry 17
ordinal data 50, 51, 60
OSCE *see* objective structured
clinical examination (OSCE)
overdose risk assessment 30
Oxford Textbook of Psychiatry
106

P

p, value 63, 64
panic, cognitive model 14
parametric statistics 51
paranoid ideas, differential
diagnosis 116
parietal lobe function 40–41
past papers 84
patient interviews 103, 125–128
patient management problems
(PMPs) 2, 4, 131–139
requirements 132
techniques 132–134
treatment resistant depression
136–138
web-based resources 135
Pearson correlation coefficient
60
personality descriptions, in IPA
123
personality disorder, differential
diagnosis 116
phobic disorders 30, 104
physical examination 103, 107

PMPs *see* patient management problems (PMPs)
The Pocket Guide to Critical Appraisal 46
positive predictive value (PPV) 55, 67
postnatal depression 42
post-test odds 67
post-test probability 67
power calculation 71
PPV (positive predictive value) 55, 67
practical skills 30, 35
pragmatic trials 72
predictive validity 70
premorbid personality 34
preparation 3, 5
  essays 84, 85
  IPA *see* individual patient assessment (IPA)
  MCQ exams 18–19
present state examination 128–130
pre-test odds 55–56, 67
pre-test probability 68
prioritisation 8
probability 74–75
prognosis 118–119
progress reviews 8
PSE (present state examination) 128–130
Psychiatric Bulletin 84
'psychodynamic formulation', in IPA 122
psychology 11, 17
psychometric tests 117
psychopathology 17

psychopharmacology 17
psychotherapy
  clinical topics MCQ paper 17
  exploratory 89–91
  OSCE 34
psychotic symptoms 30, 128–129
publication bias 76, 78
punctuality 105

Q
Q statistic 79
qualitative studies 80
questionnaires, screening and diagnosis 96

R
random effects modelling 80
randomisation procedure 71
randomised controlled trials (RCTs) 70–73
range 50, 60
rank sum tests (Wilcoxon) 51, 60
rapid tranquillisation 35
ratio data 50, 60
RCTs (randomised controlled trials) 70–73
recall bias 64
receptive dysphasia 41
referencing (essays) 99
relative risk 75
relative risk reduction (RRR) 73
reliability (in clinical studies) 68–69
research ethics 72
research methods 17, 48–49
resources 10–11

web-based *see* web-based
   resources
revision courses 5, 18
Revision Notes in Psychiatry 10
revision strategies 7–12
  condensing information
    9–10, 19
  courses 5, 18
  environmental factors 8
  learning styles 7–9
  OSCE 32–35
  resources 10–11, 46–47
    web-based *see* web-based
    resources
  timetables 3, 6, 8, 18
revision texts 10–11, 46–47
revision timetables 3, 6, 8, 18
risk assessment 42
  overdose 30
  suicide/self-harm 34, 126
Royal College of Psychiatrists
  curricula components 3
  website 2
RRR (relative risk reduction) 73

S

sample population, definition
  63
sampling procedure 49
Scheffe test 61
schizophrenia 91–97
  differential diagnosis 116
  IPA 104, 113, 126
  ISQ 13
  mock clinical exams 102
  OSCE 34
scoring schemes 14–17, 31
screening and diagnosis 66–70

questionnaires 96
selection bias 63, 64
selective serotonin re-uptake
  inhibitors (SSRIs) 37
self-harm 34
serialistic learning style 7
single case studies 80
social sciences 17
Spearman rank correlation
  coefficient 60
specificity 66–67
speech functions assessment 41
sponsors 3
SSRIs 37
standard deviation 50, 60, 61
standard error 61
stations (in OSCE) 28–30
statistical power 65–66, 71
statistical significance 63
statistical terms 60–62, 62–66,
  71
statistical tests 50–52, 60–62
  see also specific tests
statistics, basic sciences MCQ
  paper 17
Statistics with Confidence 46
stress (candidate, exam-related)
  4, 22
structured management plans
  118
study groups 9
study leave 5
subject bias 64
subject spotting 19
substance misuse
  assessment/management 34
suicide 136

risk assessment 34, 126
summary effect size 79
summary notes 9–10, 19
surveys 80
survival analysis (Kaplan Meier) 62
symptom clustering 109–110
systematic reviews 76–80

T
tables 99
target population, definition 62
TCADs 37
terminology 23–24
   see also specific topics
textbooks 10–11, 46–47
thyroid function tests 118
time management 8
topical issues 84
travel (to exams) 5
'true' questions 20–21, 23

t-tests 51, 60, 61
Type I error 65
Type II error 65

V
validity 69–70
variance 50
visual fields assessment 41

W
web-based resources 2
   essay writing 87
   MCQ exam 11
   OSCE 32
   PMPs 135
Wilcoxon rank sum tests 51, 60
writing legibility 98, 99

Z
Z test 78